Psycholog

Evaluating Mental Health Practice

With the emphasis in the 1980s on effectiveness and efficiency in health services, evaluation of practice was increasingly important. This was particularly true of mental health, where many practices were poorly evaluated and therefore might have been of questionable validity.

Originally published in 1987, this book reviews the state of evaluative research of mental health programmes at the time, showing how practices can be evaluated and hence improved. A multidisciplinary group of authors, covering psychiatry, clinical psychology, psychiatric nursing, social work and other 'therapies', describe previous studies and applications in each discipline, before detailing a case study of their own evaluative work. The book will still have something to offer all professionals concerned with improving the quality of their work in the mental health area.

Evaluating Mental Health Practice

Methods and applications

Edited by
Derek Milne

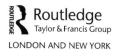
Routledge
Taylor & Francis Group

LONDON AND NEW YORK

First published in 1987
by Croom Helm Ltd

This edition first published in 2015 by Routledge
27 Church Road, Hove BN3 2FA

and by Routledge
711 Third Avenue, New York, NY 10017

Routledge is an imprint of the Taylor & Francis Group, an informa business

A Library of Congress record exists under ISBN: 0709946260

ISBN: 978-1-138-84943-3 (hbk)
ISBN: 978-1-315-72558-1 (ebk)
ISBN: 978-1-138-84944-0 (pbk)

Evaluating Mental Health Practice

Methods and Applications

Edited by Derek Milne

CROOM HELM
London • New York • Sydney

Croom Helm Ltd, Provident House,
Burrell Row, Beckenham, Kent, BR3 1AT
Croom Helm Australia, 44-50 Waterloo Road,
North Ryde, 2113, New South Wales

Published in the USA by
Croom Helm
in association with Methuen, Inc.
29 West 35th Street
New York, NY 10001

British Library Cataloguing in Publication Data

Milne, Derek
    Evaluating mental health practice: methods
    and applications.
    1. Mental health services — Great Britain
    — Evaluation
    I. Title
    362.2′0941   RA790.7.G7
    ISBN 0-7099-4626-0

Library of Congress Cataloging-in-Publication Data

Evaluating mental health practice.

    Includes bibliographies and index.
    1. Mental health services — Evaluation. 2. Community
mental health services — Evaluation. I. Milne, Derek,
1949–   . [DNLM: 1. Evaluation Studies. 2. Mental
Health Services. WM 30 E926]
RA790.5.E83   1987   362.2′028′7   87-19934
ISBN 0-7099-4626-0

Printed and bound in Great Britain
by Billing & Sons Limited, Worcester.

Contents

To Judy Milne

Acknowledgements

Edited books are notoriously difficult things to produce, and several people deserve special mention for helping me to complete this one. First and foremost amongst my helpers has been my wife, to whom the book is dedicated. She has generously allowed me space and time to beaver away on the seemingly endless editorial tasks. She has also tidied up some of my thinking and quite a bit of my English. General inspiration to grapple with the 'scientist-practitioner' approach came initially from Keith Turner (Leicester) and was then continued by my subsequent district psychologists, Iain Burnside (Wakefield) and Roger Paxton (Northumberland). Many people have contributed in general ways to my efforts along the way and I would like to pick out for special thanks Mike Corp, Charles Burdett, Ray Meddis, John Hall, Peter Salmon, Brian Stanley, Stephen Morley and Sheila Sharkey. Valuable comments on drafted chapters were received from David Parkin, Anne Broadhurst and Gail Bernstein. Secretarial support has been provided by Eileen Greaves and Stella Dickinson.

Last, but most crucial of all, I would like to thank all the contributors for their participation in this project, and extend my gratitude to Tim Hardwick for making it all possible.

Contributors

Philip J. Barker, RNMH,
Clinical Nurse Consultant,
Tayside Area Clinical
Psychology Department,
Royal Dundee Liff Hospital,
Dundee DD2 5NF,
Scotland, UK

Gail S. Bernstein, PhD,
Director, Adult Services,
John F Kennedy Child
Development Center; and
Assistant Professor,
University of Colorado
School of Medicine,
Box C234, 4200 E 9th
Avenue,
Denver, Colorado 80262,
USA

Judith Burgess,
MB, MRCPsych,
Senior Registrar,
Oxford Regional Health
Authority, UK

David Edwards BA, DipAT,
RATH, Senior Art
Therapist, Wakefield Health
Authority Mental Health
Services; and Course Tutor,
Art Therapy Training
Programme, The University
of Sheffield, 85 Wilkinson
Street, Sheffield S10 2GJ,
UK

Ian R.H. Falloon, MD,
DPM, MRCPsych,
Consultant Physician
(Mental Health),
Buckingham Hospital,
High Street, Buckingham
MK18 1NU, UK

Eileen Gambrill, PhD,
Professor, School of Social
Welfare, University of
California, Berkeley,
California 94720, USA

Roger Grainger, PhD,
Chaplain, Stanley Royd
Hospital, Wakefield, West
Yorkshire WF1 4DQ, UK

Peter Higson, Dip Clin Psych,
PhD, Course Tutor to North
Wales In-service Training
Course in Clinical
Psychology; and Principal
Clinical Psychologist, North
Wales Hospital, Denbigh,
Clwyd LL16 5SS, UK

Sheila McLees, BA,
Research Psychologist,
Buckingham Mental Health
Service, Buckingham, UK

Derek Milne, Dip Clin Psych,
PhD, Regional Tutor in
Clinical Psychology,

Northumberland Psychology
Services, Otterburn House,
East Cottingwood, Morpeth
NE61 2NU, UK

Margaret Nicol, MPhil, Dip
COT, Senior Lecturer in
Occupational Therapy,
Queen Margaret College,
Clerwood Terrace,
Edinburgh EH12 8TS,
Scotland, UK

David Skidmore, MSc, PhD,
RMN, FE Teachers Cert,
RCNT, Senior Lecturer,
Department of Applied
Community Studies,
Manchester Polytechnic,
799 Wilmslow Road,
Didsbury, Manchester
M20 8RR, UK

Greg Wilkinson, MRCP,
MRCPsych, Senior Lecturer,
General Practice Research
Unit, Institute of Psychiatry,
London, UK

Part One:
Introduction

1

Evaluating Mental Health Practice: an Introduction

Derek Milne

1.1 AIMS AND STRUCTURE OF THE BOOK

(a) Aims

Evaluation is concerned with judging the merit of something. In order to make that judgement it is essential to have a clear idea of what is being attempted. If we wished, for instance, to evaluate a psychiatric hospital we might judge it in terms of the proportion of patients who were successfully discharged. This outcome would need to be defined clearly and objectively, in terms of such factors as the services provided to sustain ex-patients in the community and the amount of time they have stayed out of hospital.

As this book deals with evaluation it is only fitting that we also have a clear idea of our goals before proceeding any further. Broadly speaking, the aim of this book is to encourage and enable mental health practitioners to do more and better evaluations of their work. It should prove to be a resourceful 'handbook'. As 'outcome data', therefore, we would hope to find that readers had undertaken evaluations which they had previously avoided, perhaps for want of such things as relevant research ideas and methods. We would also like to anticipate that those practitioners who have already undertaken evaluations of their work will benefit from this book in terms of enhancing their research skills. Although we don't propose to evaluate these aims objectively, we trust that readers will be helped to make their own evaluations of the book by this statement of goals.

1

(b) Structure

In order to pursue these goals we have designed a book that has a definite bias towards detailed and practical examples of evaluative research. Practitioners from the main mental health professions have contributed these examples, so that your own discipline (or something fairly close to it) should be represented.

We have, therefore, a wide range of practical illustrations to facilitate your involvement in good evaluative research. They cover work carried out in psychiatric and mental handicap hospitals, as well as in community settings. The programmes subjected to evaluation include a diversity of therapeutic approaches, and the assessments of these efforts are based on an equally varied range of measures and research methods.

This rich menu is unified by a recurring emphasis on the use of research methods as the best means of addressing practical problems in the mental health service. Thus the relevant experimental literature is reviewed critically and examples are provided which incorporate those features of rigorous experimental design that can be achieved in complex research settings. The limitations these can place on the results are acknowledged, but the tone is constructive; that is, focusing on how we might do a better evaluation next time around. Throughout we are reminded that such evaluations are fundamentally educative — we can all learn to be more effective clinicians because the results can serve as corrective feedback, enhancing the good practices and diminishing the bad.

The remainder of this chapter introduces and discusses evaluative research from a number of angles. We are interested first of all in defining our terms and in considering who gets involved in evaluative research. We also discuss why such research is conducted, before concluding with a section distinguishing the different types of research.

The second chapter is devoted to the problems encountered by practitioners. We try to suggest solutions to these obstacles and more generally aim to promote a constructive tone.

Part Two of the book consists of ten chapters by a wide range of mental health practitioners. These chapters review some of the research and practical issues that have concerned members of various disciplines, and provide details of the authors' own evaluation work. The aim is to give a more complete account of this work than is normally available, so as to help you to formulate your own evaluations. Each chapter is preceded by a brief summary, indicating the general nature of the evaluation study and the client group. The summaries are intended to link successive chapters, for those who wish to read from cover to cover; and to help those who just wish to 'dip in' to one or two chapters to judge the relevance of each contribution to their own interests. A simple chapter structure has been adopted, based on an alphabetical ordering of the mental health disciplines that have contributed. We therefore begin with art therapy and proceed through to social work.

Part Three is the concluding chapter. An attempt is made to review the main themes of the book and to preview some of the emerging trends in mental health evaluation. It will hopefully serve as the springboard to develop your own evaluative research efforts.

1.2 WHAT IS EVALUATIVE RESEARCH?

We all make evaluative judgements about health-related matters, and we always have. Skimming through a biography of Florence Nightingale one finds, for instance, that she wrote in 1845 that 'I saw a poor woman die before my eyes this summer because there was nothing but fools to sit up with her, who poisoned her as much as if they had given her arsenic' (Woodham-Smith, 1980, p. 55).

On the other hand Stekel, a colleague of Freud's, judged his own interventions more favourably. He described his psychoanalysis of a 35-year-old woman with depression and stated that 'the condition speedily improved after treatment' (Stekel, 1923, p. 194). Similar evaluations are to be found littering the pages of the early health literature.

However, evaluations that are based on more scientific methods are a more recent phenomenon. The most common term for this approach is 'evaluative research'. Unlike the evaluations of Stekel or Nightingale, this approach requires more systematic and rigorous care before arriving at a judgement concerning the worth of a therapy. Stekel's patient, he noted in passing, 'attributed the improvement to a water cure she underwent during the treatment' (p. 194). This alternative explanation for her cure did not change his evaluation, though, since he recognised that 'we are our patients' friends as long as they need us. When they are well again their cure is always due to something else' (p. 194). In discussing a case of hysteria, Freud himself noted how 'it still strikes me as strange that the case histories I write should read like short stories and that, as one might say, they lack the serious stamp of science' (Breuer and Freud, 1974, p. 231).

The 'stamp of science' has only latterly imposed itself on evaluations of therapeutic programmes. Holland (1983) traces the change in evaluative methods back to the nineteenth century, beginning with the collection and analysis of population data. Epidemics, birth and childhood mortality, along with many other problems, placed an increasing pressure on governments to quantify the extent of health problems and to develop therapies. At this stage, however, evaluative research methods were still weak, allowing governments and psychoanalysts alike to ascribe improvements to their efforts, when there was evidence to the contrary. For example, in the case of mortality and other indications of population health it turned out on more rigorous evaluation that improvements in environmental factors alone were responsible for the healthier statistics (McKeown and Lowe, 1966).

(a) Definition

Evaluative research, then, is something different from the clinical judgements of therapists or the simple cause–effect interpretation of population statistics. Many authors have provided definitions of evaluative research which clarify this difference. They all emphasise that it refers to the use of research methods for the purposes of judging the extent to which a therapeutic programme accomplishes its goals. As Weiss (1972) has pointed out, this involves the four central features of measurement, outcomes, explicit goals, and judging the programme's worth. Suchman (1967) adds a strongly scientific emphasis on determining whether the outcomes are attributable to the programme, or to other factors in the patient's life. He also requires that evaluative research provides a description and standardisation of the programme. Taking these points in chronological order, evaluative research is therefore the process of:

(1) identifying and defining the programme's goals;
(2) analysing the problems which the programme must face;
(3) describing and standardising the programme;
(4) measuring the amount of change that occurs;
(5) determining by the methods of experimental research the extent to which change is attributable to the programme; and
(6) assessing the relative effectiveness of modified programmes.

These, then, are the defining characteristics of evaluative research. They subsume a great diversity of approaches in each of the six areas listed above, as we shall see later. For example, the 'amount of change' may be considered clinically in terms of attitudes, understanding, coping skills or symptomatic relief, amongst many other possible programme goals. It may be measured by self-report questionnaires, medical examination, direct observation or archival statistics, along with a multitude of alternatives. Ultimately, though, the evaluation itself will be judged by the scientific criteria concerning systematic measurement. Only with acceptable standards of measurement could we infer that a programme had achieved its goals.

(b) 'Evaluative' research and 'basic' research

History may again help us to clarify another recurring issue, namely the distinction between 'basic' (or 'pure', 'traditional', 'laboratory') research and evaluative (or 'applied', 'intervention', 'field') research. Cochrane (1972) also goes back to the nineteenth century in order to locate a division between the two research traditions. It was then, he suggests, that the British science establishment divided itself into 'pure' and 'applied'. He recounts the strong tradition at Cambridge favouring the former. Moreover, he was advised by the most distinguished people that the best pure research should be 'utterly useless', so exaggerating the divide between the two traditions.

The general utility of research data is only one criterion for distinguishing evaluative from basic research. Others include the use of evaluative research data to make decisions and ask questions about specific programmes; to judge the quality of a programme against some pre-stated goals; and the pursuit of evaluative research in 'real' action settings as opposed to laboratories. Table 1.1 presents a summary of those and related distinctions.

These basic differences often have profound implications for the nature of the research that takes place. For instance, in basic research one might select subjects on the basis of testing a scientific theory. In contrast, clients in programmes that are subjected to evaluative research will participate because of a clinical problem. The questions asked in each case are therefore likely to differ considerably. The answers in the case of basic research are typically publishable contributions to a body of knowledge, whereas in evaluative research the answer is usually an attempt at improving assessment and therapy. Because the latter occurs in the 'messy' (or uncontrollable) context of one particular hospital or clinic it usually falls short of the more rigorous standards of basic research and is thus unpublishable.

Table 1.1: Some of the typical distinctions drawn between basic and evaluative research (compiled from Popham, 1975; Suchman, 1967)

Factor	'Basic' research	'Evaluative' research
1. Purpose of research	To build theories and improve understanding	To make decisions and improve programmes
2. Applicability of findings	Widely applicable	Results only directly relevant to same programme and setting
3. Value of research	To establish 'truth'	To improve worth of programme
4. Measurement	Standardised instruments; rigorous control; scientific standards essential (e.g. randomisation)	Ragbag of measuring tools; control very difficult to achieve; scientific standards desirable
5. Topics	Anything	Socially important phenomena
6. Judgement	Eschewed	Integral
7. Research consumers	Secondary, not identified	Primary
8. Politics	An improper consideration	A necessary and important consideration
9. Replicability	Important hallmark	Neither important nor possible
10. Setting	Not treated as significant; highly controlled	Essential aspect; control very limited
11. Publication	Major academic goal of research	Uncommon and secondary

Publication is made even less likely by the variety of unstandardised ways that arise of measuring programmes. But while publication is an important academic goal, it is not usually a priority in evaluative research.

As a consequence these differences tend to produce a literary world that is detached from the realities faced by clinicians in the 'field'. Pejorative terms such as 'ivory tower' research are likely to be used by practitioners exasperated by the seemingly irrelevant pursuits of academics. Figure 1.1 caricatures this perspective. It shows the academic ivory tower high up in the clouds. There sits a white-coated ('pure') researcher absorbed in 'Skinner-box' investigations of equally pure-bred laboratory rats behaving at 70 per cent of their free-feeding weight. He is also absorbed with a book which tells him how to prepare the resulting publication. The only visible context of his search for truth are other ivory tower inhabitants.

Perhaps the academics, for their part, may tend to regard evaluative researchers as 'the drones of the research fraternity, technicians drudging away on dull issues and compromising their integrity out in the corrupt world' (Weiss, 1972, p. 9).

Bolstering such extreme perceptions of basic research are reviews of the published literature relating to clinical work. Agras and Berkowitz (1980), for example, studied two major behaviour therapy journals. They found that their sample of over 200 articles contained less than 1 per cent concerned with the field efficacy of behaviour therapy, and 0 per cent dealing with disseminating methods to practitioners and programmes. This from a movement whose 'main contributions have been to advance research methods and to implement many of these developments in the field' (p. 476)!

(c) The continuum between basic and evaluative research

It is clear that basic researchers produce the great majority of published work. However, this does not necessarily serve as a hard and fast distinction between them and the evaluative researchers. We have already pointed to (Table 1.1) some reasons why the latter might not publish, even though they may be conducting systematic research approximating closely to the standards of basic researchers. In other respects the clear distinctions we made in Table 1.1 also begin to disappear on

Figure 1.1: A caricature of basic research: the 'Ivory Tower'

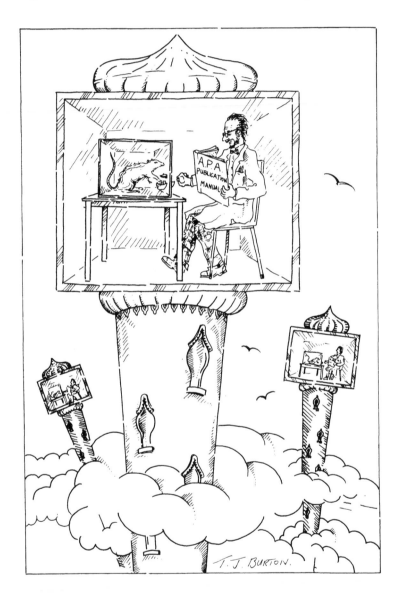

closer scrutiny. Buss (1975), for one, has drawn attention to the value-laden activities of basic researchers: choosing what to study, amongst other factors, is shaped by the values of the culture in which the scientist works. The increasing rigour of evaluative research has also thrown doubt on the distinctions raised earlier. In this respect Baer (1979) refers to recent developments in practitioners' research skills. From having been rebuffed by their academic colleagues because they knew too little, they have latterly, he asserts, been rebuffed for advancing their experimental sophistication and getting to know too much.

One plausible reason for this development has been the evaluative researchers' need to know their experimental methodology 'inside out' in order to cope with the demands of a very difficult setting (Weiss, 1972). In turn, this has led to considerable refinements in research methods. The work of Campbell and Stanley (1963) is perhaps the first real landmark in this development. They argued for the use of 'quasi-experimental' research designs when true experimental designs were impossible. To guide the practitioner they listed those factors that might limit the results, and described research methods which would minimise these limitations. Their reasoning was that although quasi-experimental research designs were less efficient than their thoroughbred relatives, the 'true' designs, they were nonetheless capable of testing out ideas, of proving them *wrong*.

Since scientific logic tells us that no number of perfectly executed experiments could ever prove an idea to be right, then imperfect attempts to prove them wrong were to be encouraged, even if these included 'weak' research designs.

The second major improvement in research methods that were suited to the practitioner came with the single-case experimental design. This allowed the clinician to treat each individual client as an experiment, taking a baseline assessment of the presenting problem before intervening, then periodically re-assessing the problem to determine which therapeutic variables were responsible for any change in the problem. The nature of the experimental design allowed the clinician to treat each client as his or her own control, so attaining scientific respectability (Hersen and Barlow, 1976).

It is therefore becoming increasingly difficult to distinguish between basic and evaluative research on the grounds of experimental sophistication alone. This has led to the view that the many different kinds of research that occur can best be regarded as points on a continuum, rather than containing clear-cut distinctions. In this vein, Suchman (1967) has talked of evaluation research as a 'bridge' between pure and applied research. That is, as using the best available methods and theories from pure experimentation and testing them out in applied settings, such as programmes. Similarly, Agras and Berkowitz (1980) have enumerated the different kinds of research that occur, ranging from clinical observations and uncontrolled evaluations through to long-term, randomised and controlled evaluative research studies. Along this continuum we have gradations in experimental rigour in relation to variations in other factors, such as the research topic or context.

To cut through this continuum and try to demark these subtle variations is bound to be 'disproved' by studies that repeatedly fail to conform to any such simple division as 'basic' versus 'evaluative' research.

In conclusion, evaluative research can be difficult to distinguish from basic research simply on the basis of experimental rigour or sophistication. On the other hand, the goals and purposes of evaluative research are distinctive, namely to help people by improving therapeutic programmes. We have argued that, far from there being a clear boundary between the two research traditions, there is a continuum along which the many diverse forms of research might be placed. Improvements in the methods of practitioners (e.g. quasi-experimental research designs; single-subject experiments) and a growing public emphasis on accountability have facilitated this transition.

This view has important implications for those working in health settings. It indicates that, far from there simply being a rare breed of scientists who conduct evaluations, all members of a service can contribute. This is so because it is not essential that every evaluation is always rigorous and precise. Rather, we can view each evaluation as a step towards the next more careful evaluation, both in terms of the individual practitioner and in terms of the programme. We can all make valuable contributions to this process of successive approximation to basic research standards. In so doing we are more likely to develop our service than if we do nothing, for instance because the research requirements are pitched at unattainably high levels. As Campbell (1969) has put it, 'we must do the best we can with what is available to us' (p. 411). Not only can this 'experimental' orientation help us to develop our programmes, it can also facilitate the professional development of therapist skills. This is because our evaluations can provide feedback to us on the way we work, and from such information we can learn to be better therapists. It also follows that by participating in research we are putting ourselves in the position to learn more about experimentation.

1.3 WHO DOES EVALUATIVE RESEARCH?

Another way of summarising the developmental view outlined above is to say that evaluative research is what interested practitioners do. In this sense members of any professional group in any setting can gradually evolve relevant research skills. The data from this research orientation can then serve as corrective feedback, reducing the ineffective elements of a programme while increasing the more effective ones. This may encourage researchers to do more and better evaluations.

The use of carefully gathered data is, of course, only one impetus to change. Over recent centuries we have witnessed the contributions made by visionary clergymen, guilt-ridden do-gooders and political radicals, as Freeman and Sherwood (1965) have referred to some of the major forces acting on health programmes. Such agents do not do evaluative research, although they probably make profound evaluations.

In fact, relatively few people do undertake evaluative research. The health field is notable for the number of people in favour of doing it and the few who actually try (Zusman and Ross, 1969). Even those whose professional status might force this approach upon them seem reluctant to get involved. Campbell (1969) describes programme administrators in this light, drawing attention to some of the factors that influence their research activities. Principal amongst these is their commitment to the efficacy of a programme in advance of any data. Then when data are considered they are gathered in ways that maximise the likelihood that their programme will look good. One illustration Campbell offers is that of 'grateful testimonials' which exploit human courtesy and gratitude to assure the administrator of a favourable evaluation. In the absence of any other information these data will often be sufficient to ossify the programme in whatever favoured shape it is in. In contrast, Campbell describes the 'experimental' administrator. These people have not committed themselves dogmatically to the programme in advance of the evidence. Rather, they set up a service on the best available information in response to an important social problem. They undertake as a matter of routine good practice to evaluate systematically this first attempt at the service. The inevitable strengths and weaknesses that emerge are not seen as criticisms or personal failure, but as guidance on how to develop the programme. The administrator is behaving like an impartial scientist, looking at the evidence before judging the success or otherwise of the service. Their commitment is to this style of reform, not to a particular therapeutic approach. It follows that they are not threatened by a careful analysis of the programme.

It would be naive, however, to imagine that we might simply choose to become one of Campbell's 'experimental' practitioners. There are many good reasons for adopting other survival styles in health services, some of which we will discuss shortly. Nonetheless, some members of all the health service groups do at times conduct evaluative research. Our emphasis in this book will be on understanding and developing their style of work, since they must have found ways of adopting the 'experimental' mode. Another term for this work orientation that has wide currency is that of 'scientist–practitioner' (Barlow, Hayes and Nelson, 1984). In this book our emphasis is on moving from a practitioner base into research. For this reason we will prefer the expression 'practitioner–scientist'.

In conclusion, evaluative research is carried out by a very wide variety of health service staff, despite formidable obstacles. The contents of this book testify to this wide interest. These people would seem to have adopted an 'experimental' or 'practitioner–scientist' approach to their work, one which requires them systematically to evaluate what they do, so as to improve the service to their clients. The research continuum, discussed earlier, makes it possible for practitioners with limited research training to develop relevant skills and programmes.

However, breadth of interest is not matched by depth: relatively few people actually undertake evaluative research.

1.4 WHY DO EVALUATIVE RESEARCH?

Given the many difficulties that attend systematic programme evaluation one must ask why anyone should bother. In this final section we consider some of the reasons for starting and sustaining an involvement in evaluative research.

(a) Clinical feedback

One fundamental motive for doing research is that it offers us an objective basis for developing our services and skills. Evaluation data can provide us with 'feedback' on our programme and our own therapeutic skills. This is necessary since, as the old adage goes, there is no learning without feedback.

This is to be contrasted, in Campbell's (1969) terms, to the 'trapped' practitioner, who is blindly committed to a programme and hence unable to test out their service truly. It also follows that they do not facilitate their own learning as clinicians, since they restrict information that might tell them when they've got it wrong. Equally, the clients are subjected to a misguided programme run by the unnecessarily restricted skills of such practitioners. As Barlow et al. (1984) suggest, such a state of affairs is ethically unjustifiable: without careful evaluation how can a practitioner know if a programme benefits its clients?

(b) Accountability

Human services have entered the era of accountability. Public attitudes, financial constraints and legislative mandates have increasingly demanded that programmes produce evidence that they work (Hawkins, Fremouw and Reitz, 1981). This is becoming true of even the most plausible and expensive interventions. One striking illustration comes from a careful evaluation of coronary care units. When compared with the traditional at-home approach no advantage was demonstrated in admission to costly units (Mather, Pearson, Read et al., 1971).

Because of such questions about the relative value of different therapeutic programmes, the United States Senate introduced legislation in 1980 and 1981 requiring the clear

13

demonstrations of the safety, efficacy and appropriateness of various programmes before reimbursement was forthcoming (Barlow *et al.*, 1984).

(c) Decision-making

Evaluative research is committed to the principle of utility, and particularly to influencing decision-making. If it has no such influence it is an exercise in organisational futility (Weiss, 1972), although the individual researcher may well benefit. The decisions that may be influenced include those concerning the continuation of a programme, changes in practices and procedures, changes in location or clientele, resource allocation between competing programmes and the acceptance or rejection of a given programme approach. If practitioners have a concern for such questions they may be more interested in evaluative research as a means of influencing decisions that directly affect them.

(d) Enhance science

Many principles relevant to clinical problems have been refined in laboratory research. The big question, Baer (1979) asserts, is whether these principles have *generality*; to what extent do they hold up across different settings, clients and problems? He sees this generality question as the ultimate test of any 'pure' research findings, for unless they are robust enough to withstand applications in the real world they have little clinical value. However, if they do withstand such examinations they can extend or refine the scientific principles.

(e) Avoidance and escape

In addition to the foregoing laudable reasons for doing research, clinicians will be aware that their behaviour is often controlled by aversive means. Evaluative research, like phobic behaviour, may be determined by the avoidance of unpleasant consequences. Illustrations are the use of an evaluation to postpone a decision that has aversive consequences. In this sense appointing a large committee to report on the future of a programme

14

ensures longevity and promotes avoidance. We can also escape any responsibility for decision-making by sponsoring an evaluation, thereby allowing the results (or the evaluators) to shoulder the consequences of an unpleasant decision. Brownescombe-Heller (1984) develops this theme by discussing fear of failure and fear of success amongst psychologists. She suggests we can tell them apart because in the former the research is sabotaged early on; whereas in the 'fear of success' state we proceed smoothly until the end is in sight, whereupon self-sabotage occurs. Typical sabotage rationalisations include: 'I don't have an adequate control group', 'it's all been said before' and 'research is nothing but an ego trip'.

(f) Social reinforcement

I alluded earlier to the 'ivory tower' orientation to research in which the ideal was that the best research was 'utterly useless' (Cochrane, 1972, p. 9). While this may well have precluded scientists from the more obvious commercial rewards that may now attend some evaluative research, it is not to say that their work had no social consequences. Cochrane highlights one when he goes on to point out that 'useless' research was 'U', was approved by the Medical Research Council and was endorsed by one's colleagues.

As Salmon (1983) has pointed out, social consequences follow all sorts of research activity. Publications, conference papers, promotion, and general social accolades are some of the more obvious positive reinforcers. There are also, of course, more aversive consequences, such as papers being rejected, or colleagues' judgements that our research is an idle extravagance. In contrast, direct work with clients is always pressing and socially valid. This behavioural perspective suggests that these consequences are crucial determinants of our involvement in evaluative research, rather than some kind of idealistic 'thirst for knowledge'.

1.5 TYPES OF EVALUATIVE RESEARCH

The traditional focus of evaluation studies is the result or 'outcome' produced by a programme. This is, however, only one possible concern, and several other ways of assessing programmes have been applied. We will now briefly review these approaches, broadly following the work of Suchman (1967). Some published illustrations of these approaches will be provided, and further examples follow later in this book.

(a) Effort

The basic question one asks in an effort evaluation concerns the activities that take place in a programme and the related resources and energy invested in those activities. It is assumed that increased effort correlates positively with increased efficiency. Records of the unit's resources (staffing, equipment, facilities, financing, etc.) and their utilisation (staff-to-patient interaction, use of equipment, etc.) provide the relevant data.

Effort is one of the easiest dimensions of a programme to evaluate and it can be a useful indicator of what is being done about a problem. Also, effort is a necessary condition for efficiency, although clearly not sufficient in the absence of the requisite clinical skills. Thus, a mental health programme may have as its goals the alleviation of certain symptoms for a given proportion of a population. To establish that all the staff work very hard in order to see all these clients would (crudely speaking) represent an effort evaluation. It does not necessarily follow that all this hectic effort actually achieves the desired symptom reduction in clients, although some effort will undoubtedly be necessary. If the amount of effort has increased over some earlier assessment we would expect, but could not guarantee, better programme results.

(b) Outcome

An outcome evaluation focuses on the effects or results of a programme. It addresses such questions as who benefits and by how much?; was the programme goal achieved and did any change occur? Outcome evaluations are the most fundamental way of determining the effectiveness of a service. They tend to provide the ultimate answers required by funders, practitioners or users about whether a programme 'works', as well as providing a pivot around which all other types of evaluation turn.

16

'Effort' evaluations, for instance, need to be related to 'outcome' if we are to demonstrate that changes in effort are worthwhile. In this sense outcome evaluations take us away from the traditional emphasis on the simple existence of a service as an end in itself, towards a consideration of the service as a means to an end, namely improving programme effectiveness. This is widely accepted as the most essential type of evaluation and there is a trend towards this and away from other ways of judging programmes (Lloyd, 1983).

Two basic questions may be posed in outcome evaluations. The first and least important of these is whether someone changed through exposure to a programme. This is a weak form of evaluation because small but statistically significant results may be obtained, although there is little practical improvement. The second and more important question asks whether the client changed enough to produce an improvement in everyday functioning (Kazdin, 1977). Evaluations of this type are referred to as 'goal attainment' measures. To apply such a measure one has to establish the current 'baseline' level of a clinical problem then specify with the client some valuable goals. These are then reviewed at different stages in treatment, as illustrated in psychiatric rehabilitation by Stanley (1984). Lloyd (1983) has reviewed five goal attainment measures.

(c) Process

A more traditional focus in programme evaluation has been on the number of clients served and the range of services provided. Accounts which detail such factors are predominant in the literature, but they are really more descriptive than evaluative, saying little about the related outcome or effort.

Another form of process evaluation which is much more penetrating and far less common deals with the relationship between parts of a programme and their individual or collective outcome. This approach examines the attributes of a programme so as to seek out those factors that make it more or less successful. The basic question it asks is: 'what goes on here?' To refer forward to the discussion on 'fuzzy' accounts of a programme's ingredients, process evaluations can address the issue of what exactly is happening in such events as 'counselling' or 'anxiety management'. Two ways of proceeding are either to examine one programme element in detail, or to compare its relative effectiveness with another component. The unifying concern is in identifying by *which* means *what* results are achieved.

Zusman and Ross (1969) have distinguished four methods of undertaking process evaluations. They are: inviting an 'expert' to audit the programme records; examination of the conditions of clients after treatment; assessing the proficiency of staff; and direct observation of staff activities. An interesting example of the latter has been provided by Sanson-Fisher and Jenkins (1978), who observed staff–client interactions within a social learning analysis. This indicated to them that the clients coerced the staff away from the goals of the programme, as in the clients providing 'positive attention' to staff 97 per cent of the time when they were doing the clients' chores for them! The effect was to reduce the therapeutic interactions between staff and clients, so undermining the overall programme.

This example indicates how irrelevant 'effort' evaluations could prove to be in trying to understand the value of a programme. Conversely, it suggests that sensitive evaluations of the therapeutic process may be needed to grasp what is actually happening in a programme, and hence of allowing us to make sense of any outcome results.

(d) Efficiency

Outcome evaluations can tell us whether our programme achieves its goals, and process evaluations may indicate how this is achieved. However, it is possible to have very effective programmes that are clearly understood but which are too expensive to sustain. This raises the need for 'efficiency' evaluations. These focus on the cost of obtaining programme goals and on developing less expensive alternatives. An illustration we gave earlier was the finding that specially built and staffed coronary care units were no more effective than the traditional home care method.

Programme costs include time, personnel, buildings, maintenance and so on. An 'efficient' programme would produce better outcomes for the same cost, or the same ones for less. If, for instance, we ran 1-hour groups for six clients in anxiety management, and this was just as effective in reducing avoidance behaviour as seeing clients individually for $1/2$ hour each, we'd have a three-fold increase in efficiency. Mangen, Paykel, Griffith *et al.* (1983) have given an account of efficiency evaluation. They compared the cost of outpatient appointments with a psychiatrist against the cost of a community psychiatric nurse (CPN) as the main therapist for chronic 'neurotic' clients during follow-up. Costs taken into account included the use of general practitioners (GPs), day centres, home helps, unemployment and sickness benefits, rent and rate rebates, and travel costs. The authors concluded that the CPN service was cheaper overall than outpatient appointments with the psychiatrist, and since it was also more highly regarded it could be seen as an efficient and attractive alternative to conventional practice. Yates (1985) has provided a thorough introduction to this kind of cost-effectiveness evaluation.

(e) Client satisfaction

Evaluations of efficiency are rare but increasingly evident, in contrast to assessments of client satisfaction, which have a very lengthy history. The acceptability of a service is potentially crucial, in so far as intolerable or unsatisfactory provisions will be underused, even if they are very effective or efficient (Holland, 1983).

The most common methods of evaluating client satisfaction have been reviewed by Lebow (1982). They include questionnaire surveys, complaints or statements of approval and observations or estimates of programme utilisation (e.g. promptness, dropouts, etc.). Although satisfaction can be readily measured, its relationship to other outcome indications is often puzzling. Lebow (1982) reported wide variations in correlations between client satisfaction and such indices as client- and therapist-rated clinical outcomes. More broadly, Parker and Thomas (1980) cite examples from education where the students who learned the most rated their instructors least favourably. Such findings cast doubt on what we can learn or judge from client satisfaction evaluations. Perhaps one promising way of clarifying matters is to distinguish between different aspects of satisfaction, as Wolf (1978) has done. In his analysis three dimensions are highlighted, namely the 'goals', 'procedures' and 'outcomes' of a programme. Having made this distinction, we may be well advised to study 'satisfaction' as a necessary condition for a client's use of a service.

1.6 SUMMARY AND CONCLUSIONS

The use of the scientific method to study health problems has a short history. We have used the term 'evaluative research' to refer to this approach, which essentially involves assessing by objective and systematic means the extent to which a therapeutic programme achieves its goals. Unlike the traditional 'basic' research of university laboratories, evaluative research is explicitly intended to guide us in our attempts to ameliorate clinical problems and to aid decision-making about the future developments of a programme. However, wherever applicable the rigorous standards of laboratory research are to be applied: 'evaluative research' should not, and need not, be synonymous with 'poor research'. Indeed, the demands placed on those who conduct research with 'real' subjects in 'real' settings may result in the refinement of both scientific methodology and theories, making it the envy of basic researchers.

Another major implication of the evaluative research approach is that it can and often does incorporate all the practitioners in a programme. It is thus not necessarily an exclusive role adopted by outside experts, but rather a potential aspect of the routine work of all practitioners. From this perspective it follows that we can structure evaluations of our work so that we obtain objective feedback. This can serve both to develop the skills of individual clinicians and to promote the evolution of an overall programme, so benefiting staff and clients alike. Another implication that we have drawn out in this introduction is that research skills can develop in the same way as clinical skills. This view suggests that we can all gradually acquire the necessary skills to conduct a scientific evaluation. For this reason we have adopted the term 'practitioner–scientist'. Similarly, we can develop expertise in those kinds of evaluations that most concern us in our work-place, rather than working to some idealised standard. In this sense we can conceive that under some circumstances a scientifically 'soft' client satisfaction evaluation may be more relevant and helpful than an efficiency trial. There are, then, two overlapping dimensions. One concerns the wide range of research skills that practitioner–

scientists can bring to bear on a clinical problem; and the second dimension is the wide range of research strategies that might be employed.

The essential requirement is not, therefore, a thorough undergraduate training in research methods but an 'experimental' orientation to one's work. Given this basic curiosity, some guidance and some motivation, we can acquire those research skills that are relevant to us and our work-place. This book is an attempt to encourage these conditions.

REFERENCES

Agras, W.S. and Berkowitz, R. (1980) 'Clinical Research in Behavior Therapy: Halfway There?', *Behavior Therapy, 11*, 472-87

Baer, D.M. (1979) 'On the Relation between Basic and Applied Research', in: A.C. Catania and T.A. Brigham (eds), *Handbook of Applied Behavior Analysis*, Irvington Publishers, New York

Barlow, D.H., Hayes, S.C. and Nelson, R.O. (1984) *The Scientist–Practitioner*, Pergamon Press, London

Breuer, J. and Freud, S. (1974) *Studies on Hysteria*, Penguin Books, Harmondsworth, UK

Brownescombe-Heller, M. (1984) 'PROCRAST: Why Don't Psychologists Do More Research?', *Newsletter of the British Psychological Society's Division of Clinical Psychology, 45*, 35-40

Buss, A.R. (1975) 'The Emerging Field of the Sociology of Psychological Knowledge' *American Psychologist, 30*, 988-1002

Campbell, D.T. (1969) 'Reforms on Experiments', *American Psychologist, 24*, 409-29

Campbell, D.T. and Stanley, J.C. (1963) *Experimental and Quasi-experimental Designs for Research*, Rand McNally, Chicago

Cochrane, A.L. (1972) *Effectiveness and Efficiency*, Nuffield Provincial Hospitals Trust, London

Freeman, H.E. and Sherwood, C.C. (1965) 'Research in Large-scale Intervention Programmes', *Journal of Social Issues, 21*, 11-28

Hawkins, R.P., Fremouw, W.J. and Reitz, A.L. (1981) 'A Model for Use in Designing or Describing Evaluations of Mental Health or Educational Intervention Programmes', *Behavioural Assessment, 3*, 307-24

Hersen, M. and Barlow, D.H. (1976) *Single Case Experimental Designs: Strategies for Studying Behavior Change*, Pergamon Press, New York

Holland, W.W. (ed.) (1983) *Evaluation of Health Care*, Oxford University Press, Oxford

Kazdin, A.E. (1977) 'Assessing the Clinical or Applied Importance of Behaviour Change through Social Validation', *Behaviour Modification, 1*, 427-51

Lebow, J. (1982) 'Consumer Satisfaction with Mental Health Treatment', *Psychological Bulletin, 91,* 244-59

Lloyd, M.E. (1983) 'Selecting Systems to Measure Client Outcome in Human Service Agencies', *Behavioural Assessment, 5,* 55-70

Mangen, S.P., Paykel, E.S., Griffith, J.H., Burchell, A. and Mancini, P. (1983) 'Cost-effectiveness of Community Psychiatric Nurse or Outpatient Psychiatrist Care of Neurotic Patients', *Psychological Medicine, 13,* 407-16

Mather, H.G., Pearson, W.G., Read, K.L., Shaw, K.L.Q., Steed, D.B., Thorner, G.R., Jones, M.G., Guerrier, C.J., Eraut, C.D., McHugh, P.M., Chowdhurz, N.R., Jafary, M.K. and Wallace, T.J. (1971) 'Acute Myocardial Infarction, Home and Hospital Treatment', *British Medical Journal, 3,* 334

McKeown, T. and Lowe, C.R. (1966) *An Introduction to Social Medicine,* Blackwell Scientific Publications, Oxford

Parker, R.M. and Thomas, K.R. (1980) 'Fads, Flaws, Fallacies and Foolishness in Evaluation of Rehabilitation Programmes', *Journal of Rehabilitation, 46,* 32-4

Popham, W.J. (1975) *Educational Evaluation,* Prentice-Hall, Englewood Cliffs, NJ

Salmon, P. (1983) 'Psychologists and the Community: Is Counterinfluence Enough?' *Bulletin of the British Psychological Society, 36,* 369-71

Sanson-Fisher, R. and Jenkins, H.J. (1978) 'Interaction Patterns between In-mates and Staff in a Maximum Security Institution for Delinquents', *Behavior Therapy, 9,* 703-16

Stanley, B.S. (1984) 'The Use of Goal Attainment Scaling', *Journal of Advanced Nursing, 9,* 351-6

Stekel, W. (1923) *Conditions of Nervous Anxiety and their Treatment,* Kegan Paul, London

Suchman, E.A. (1967) *Evaluative Research,* Russell Sage, New York

Weiss, C.H. (1972) *Evaluation Research,* Prentice-Hall, Englewood Cliffs, NJ

Wolf, M.M. (1978) 'Social Validity: the Case for Subjective Measurement or How Applied Behavior Analysis is Finding its Heart', *Journal of Applied Behavior Analysis, 11,* 203-14

Woodham-Smith, C. (1980) *Florence Nightingale,* Constable, London

Yates, B.T. (1985) 'Cost-effectiveness Analysis and Cost–Benefit Analysis: an Introduction', *Behavioural Assessment, 7,* 207-34

Zusman, J. and Ross, R.R. (1969) 'Evaluation of the Quality of Mental Health Services', *Archives of General Psychiatry, 20,* 352-7

2

Problems and Solutions
in Evaluation

Derek Milne

2.1   INTRODUCTION

In order to understand why so little evaluative research is
conducted we need to consider the obstacles that face practitioners. These problems are numerous, and anyone beginning
their development as a practitioner in the time-honoured
manner with a review of the relevant literature will not find
much encouragement. To begin with the titles of articles indicate that the authors have had a rough time, with references to
'turbulent settings', 'community cauldrons', 'the first 20 years
are the hardest', and innovators being eaten by dragons. If the
beginning practitioner–scientists get past these ordeals they
must then face an intimidating list of problems. Let us consider
some of the main examples by utilising the characteristic
elements of evaluative research, as described on page 5. We
follow each problem with some possible solutions, so as to
encourage a constructive tone. For illustration, we will refer to a
psychiatric day hospital in which the author was based.

2.2   IDENTIFYING GOALS

(a) Possible problems

Without clearly defined goals a programme simply cannot be
evaluated. It is meaningless to ask the basic evaluative research
questions (e.g. 'did the programme work?') without some
predetermined objective in mind. This is why this step comes
first. But as Weiss (1972) points out, goals of programmes are

often unstated or presented as 'pious platitudes' (p. 25). Freeman and Sherwood (1965) provide an amusing account of the researchers' options. They can try to guess the programme goals, and later be told that the ones selected were irrelevant; they can insist that the programme's personnel provide specific goals ('in which case the researcher should bring lots of novels to the office to read while he waits', p. 17); or they can participate in clarifying goals.

On top of the absence or ambiguity of programme goals there are numerous other obstacles. They include the unpredictable or shifting nature of programmes (changes in priorities, policy, etc.), the embedding of the service within larger organisational units (problems in 'bureaucracy', representation in decision-making meetings); and the 'unofficial' goals of programmes. To illustrate the last point, staff in a rehabilitation programme may work towards the official goal of maximising the patients' independence. However, since this entails changes in their work and may even threaten their employment, they may be forgiven if they try to keep 'official' goals vague and unattainable.

(b) Possible solutions

Identifying the goals of a programme can undoubtedly be a taxing task, but it is by no means an insuperable one. The first step is to avoid 'fuzzies'. These are vague statements of goals that everyone might applaud but few could define. Examples are that 'aggression', or 'schizophrenia', or 'anti-social behaviour', or 'personality disorder' and so on be 'reduced'. Equally, a programme may state as its goal that desirable behaviours be 'increased'. It might aim to 'develop' 'insight', or 'self-awareness' or 'personality' and so forth. Whether the aim is to increase or decrease individual characteristics they must be stated with much greater clarity and specificity. This is so because 'fuzzy' goals are too elusive for evaluation purposes: for instance, how could we agree on whether and how much 'insight' had been achieved? In this sense, 'fuzzy' goals are no better than no goals; indeed, they may be worse, as they may obscure objectives and evaluation, so retarding the programme's development.

In place of fuzzy goals we should strive for clearly stated and specific ones. We refer to these as 'performances'. These over-come the problems just mentioned and also permit us to measure programme effects objectively. Thus we may decide that the term 'insight' really boils down to a number of observable events. These may be certain kinds of statements made by clients or a range of activities they undertake as a consequence of the programme. 'Insight' for an agoraphobic may then be defined in terms of a client's stated awareness that a panic attack is only anxiety and not anything worse (e.g. impending madness). In terms of related actions we would be able to observe whether or not the individual was able to do things previously avoided, and so on. In this way 'insight' becomes a performance rather than a fuzzy: it is something we can all observe and whose occurrence we can agree upon. This paves the way to accurate measurement by changing the idiosyncratic interpretations of practitioners into scientific data.

Then, the next step is to ensure that the goals are indeed measurable. Our example of the agoraphobic's performance goals could be quantified by self-reported or practitioner-observed avoidance. We might utilise published questionnaires for this purpose or develop our own observation measure. In this manner we could measure the response of agoraphobics in our programme and evaluate the extent to which we were achieving our goals. These might be stated in quite specific terms, such as 50 per cent less avoidance after 3 months participation in the programme. After 3 months we could repeat our measuring exercise and compare this with the initial 'baseline' score and so readily determine whether our programme had achieved its goal.

In practice, goal definition is much more than an exercise in semantics and science. Rather, it is a political 'bomb' to be defused by carefully negotiating acceptable and relevant goals with both clients and staff. Both groups are likely to have an investment in the status quo and will not be eager to set in train the process of evaluation and change. There are, however, constructive ways of addressing these problems. The essential questions (such as what is to be changed, who is to be the client group and how is change to be procured) can be raised so that the evaluator can be flexible about possible goals, since this is crucial both for negotiations and sensitive measurement. The requirements of goal definition (i.e. specific performances that are measurable) must of course be adhered to and this may prove to be the main task facing the evaluator.

One helpful way of articulating possible goals, and of encouraging discussion, is to employ simple graphic accounts of programmes. An example is the Ward Atmosphere Scale (WAS; Moos, 1974). The WAS can provide a general orientation to the programme and facilitate relevant goal-setting. In our illustration from a psychiatric day hospital an initial evaluation of the clinical outcomes achieved by patients indicated that few gains were being made (Milne, 1984). We then discussed WAS profiles based on both patients' and staff opinions about the unit. These led to agreement on a number of programme changes, with resulting improvements in the ward atmosphere and in the clinical results (Milne, 1986a, b). An illustration from the WAS profile at the baseline assessment is offered in Figure 2.1.

Figure 2.1: The 'Real' (0– – –0)–'Ideal' (×——×) Discrepancy on the Ward Atmosphere Scale (WAS) for the nurses at the first baseline assessment (N=6). An asterisk denotes a statistically significant discrepancy between the 'real' and 'ideal' means.

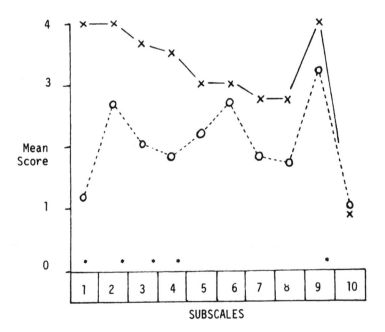

This figure shows a line for how staff actually perceived the unit (the 'real' ward) and a second for how they would like it to be (the 'ideal' ward). It can be seen that their view of the 'real' and 'ideal' wards are quite different, indicating general areas of dissatisfaction, such as in the lack of programme clarity. This figure (and those based on the patients' WAS replies, which were in fact very similar) was a great help in getting staff to clarify the programme and its goals. It is likely that they were much more willing to consider changes when possible problems were presented in this way and were based on their own opinions.

Goal attainment scaling is another promising approach. Various types of measures are available which allow practitioners to list areas in which individual clients wish to change (Lloyd, 1983). If applied routinely to all those who enter a programme then overall programme goals could be defined in terms of a summary of the individual clients' needs.

2.3. ANALYSING PROGRAMME TASKS

(a) Possible problems

Programmes usually involve several professional groups, each with their own distinctive perspective on what the programme is attempting to achieve. There are then administrators and clients with additional views, not to mention the wider social interpretation that may be placed on a programme by politicians or the general public (e.g. neighbours).

Moreover, these groups are faced with meshing the earlier problem of goal definition with their perception of the programme's tasks. To continue the earlier example, the nursing staff may formally work towards the goal of independence, whereas the local populace may oppose the resulting discharge of patients to the community. Does a programme task then become one of persuading neighbourhoods to accept ex-patients, while the 'community' is busy trying to persuade the programme that its task is to retain them?

Even leaving aside such issues, there are difficulties at the more basic level of deciding how a programme should achieve its goals: which analytic framework should prevail; and for which people (staff or patients)? Epidemiological data are not always available as a basis for planning local priorities, and even when they are, other factors may determine the direction a programme takes, as in the special interests or skills of its particular group of personnel.

The developing evaluative researcher will pay heed to these potential obstacles, or pay the price in ruined plans. The golden rule appears to be to define the specific programme tasks that are of interest, and relate these to equally specific and limited goals. Thus our rehabilitation nurses could focus on preparing a patient for discharge to the community using a given therapeutic approach, and evaluate their success in terms of a range of 'discharge' criteria. These could include systematic assessments of the efficacy of the therapy approach in helping an individual to become more independent, or analysing problems in securing acceptance of that person in the community.

(b) Possible solutions

As we have seen, the problems facing a programme can be defined in terms of clients, practitioners or wider social groups. The obvious starting place is to consider the assessment of the clients' needs as the main task facing a programme. It is against this standard that one might best determine how well a programme is succeeding.

In one sense this refers to the number of people with given needs, and in another related sense it refers to how we might best meet these needs. The way of addressing the first issue is epidemiological — we can assess samples of people to determine how many potential clients there might be in a population. An illustration is the use of the General Health Questionnaire (GHQ; Goldberg, 1978) to identify psychiatric 'cases'. This can be administered to samples of people attending other health service settings, such as general practitioners' surgeries. Various estimates can then be derived about the number of 'cases' and the general nature of their problems. This could guide decision-making about resources and types of programmes.

A second level on which this kind of survey can usefully proceed is within a sample of clients already participating in a programme. The question here is whether the existing programmes are meeting the clients' needs. To return to the earlier example, our day hospital was admitting a very wide range of people and problems. All of these people had broad needs that were addressed (food, shelter, company, activity, etc.), but they also had specific needs that were initially rarely identified. Our first task, in terms of evaluating the problems faced by the programme, was therefore to enumerate and prioritise the needs of this group. We did this by analysing their referral forms, which included considerable information about each individual's needs, then using these data to decide on changes in the contents and order of the programme. Table 2.1 provides a summary of this information. This shows that anxiety was the single most common problem identified for this group of clients. Until this time the programme had made no special provision for treating anxiety, as reflected in the ward atmosphere and the poor clinical outcomes mentioned earlier. However, by summarising and ranking problems the ground was prepared for an evaluation of the clinical tasks facing the programme.

The analysis of the referral forms also yielded information on whether the day hospital was serving its role as a 'stepping

Table 2.1: A summary of some of the information available on a group of patients (N=74) referred to the day hospital*

Problem area	Specific complaints	Percentage of those referred who had the problem
Social	Unassertive	38
	No friend	35
	Talks with difficulty	23
Occupational	Currently unemployed	100
	Lost work habit	50
	Unaware of work demands	49
	Not able to use outside agencies	45
Clinical	Diagnosis of depression	37
	Diagnosis of anxiety	63
	Dependent on staff	33
	Management problem	30
	Urinary incontinence	8
	Diagnosis of dementia	10
Demographic information	Age (mean)	50 years old
	Marital status	24% married
	Sex	65% male; 35% female
	Inpatient history	85% had been inpatients in last 6 months
	Reason for referral	23% for active treatment

*Totals exceed 100 per cent because multiple complaints were specified for each client.

stone' between inpatient and outpatient status, along with other potentially valuable guides to the problems faced by the programme (e.g. employment history, period as inpatient).

Turning to the second issue we raised, once we have clarified the clients' clinical needs there still remains the vexed question of how we might best meet those needs. Not only is it plausible that different therapeutic approaches produce different results; it is also possible that informal or non-professional sources of help are as effective as the formal agencies (Winefield, 1984; Milne and Mullin, 1987). It would seem that the best way to address these issues is by the systematic evaluation of relevant alternatives, that is by adopting the 'experimental' approach to programme development as advocated by Campbell (1969).

2.4 DESCRIBING AND STANDARDISING PROGRAMMES

(a) Possible problems

Because the practitioners who run programmes are concerned first and foremost with producing a good therapeutic effect, they will apply all kinds of interventions at a variety of times in order to achieve this outcome. Unfortunately, the dictates of helping people by whatever means may be available produces an endlessly changing programme. This is unfortunate from an evaluation standpoint, since it becomes difficult to determine what causes what and hence to evolve better ways of helping people in the future.

To consider the issue of programme change first, it is unlikely that all the important variables remain constant during a period of evaluative research. Staff may change their procedures or may be absent or be replaced. Programme users may be equally variable, influencing the content and process of events. Decisions affecting the programme may be taken and implemented, drastically altering it from the form originally studied. Not surprisingly, researchers have attempted to overcome these difficulties by establishing control over the programme (e.g. Fairweather, 1967), but more often the practitioner–scientist has very little control or influence at this organisational level.

So far we have been concerned with changes in the programme during the evaluation period. Another related problem is that descriptions of the programme at any one point in time are jeopardised by inconsistencies. These arise between a written or stated programme and what actually takes place. Table 2.2 presents the programme in our illustrative day hospital. This problem concerns at least two elements: on the one hand activities may only occur a variable proportion of the allocated time; while on the other hand their 'labels' may not correspond closely with what happens. In this sense a programme may allow an hour a day for 'anxiety management'. But the hour may be lost because of late arrivals, staff shortages in other parts of the hospital or the needs of a current intake of clients.

The second facet of programme inconsistencies is that even when stated activities do occur they may be described in terms that obscure or mislead the reader. Illustrations of 'fuzzy' terms include 'staff meetings', 'discussion groups' and 'therapeutic outings'. These may conceivably cover any range of activities. The same may be said about different therapeutic techniques, even when seemingly precise labels are applied. 'Anxiety management', for instance, usually refers to a package of techniques including progressive muscular relaxation, cognitive behaviour therapy and graded exposure *in vivo*. Different therapists from different disciplines may very well add and subtract from this package, as well as each applying the techniques somewhat differently. This is also a common problem in the wider research field. Peterson, Homer and Wonderlich (1982) reviewed some behaviour therapy studies and found that although adequate descriptions were usually provided of the outcome measures (i.e. the effects of therapy), very few studies provided adequate details of the actual therapy procedures themselves. As with other programmes this makes it very difficult to repeat the study, and so limits its usefulness.

Table 2.2: The written programme at the day hospital

Film	Drama therapy
Recreational activities	Art therapy
Handicrafts	Social skills group
Gardening	Musical appreciation
Relaxation training	Individual casework
Crossword	Anxiety management group
Dance therapy	

In summary, problems such as these make the standardisation of programmes difficult. It follows that evaluative research becomes difficult to execute, interpret or repeat.

(b) Possible solutions

Problems such as those that arise because of changes in staffing or clients have been classed as threats to the 'internal validity' of an experiment (Campbell and Stanley, 1963). They parallel such factors as history or maturation because they represent alternative explanations for the results. Thus, rather than simply attributing the outcome we achieve to the effects of our programme, we have to take into account the possibility that other changes were responsible. To illustrate, staff changes may introduce more enthusiasm or proficiency; while client changes may result in less chronicity or more motivation. These unplanned changes may well produce a more powerful effect than the deliberate programme modifications.

To overcome such threats to the internal validity of our evaluation we can alter our research design. We will discuss this broad issue more fully in section 2.5 below, but here we can focus on one design strategy that can minimise interpretation problems. We can repeatedly reassess clients, either at short intervals (e.g. monthly), or immediately before and after any changes. This allows us to estimate the effect of things such as staff changes in relation to the effect of the overall programme. Another option which is perhaps worth considering, but is often less practicable, is deliberately to manipulate an unplanned change once it has occurred, or to assess its impact under different conditions that arise naturally. For instance, consider the situation if clients from our example day hospital were in the middle of a follow-up evaluation when community psychiatric nurses (CPNs) took up posts and started visiting the clients. This represents an alternative explanation for any results we obtain, since we could not confidently exclude the effects of the CPNs' visits from those due to the programme they had completed. We might then compare two subsamples of these discharged clients, one known to be receiving CPN visits and the other not. On the hypothesis that the visits do have an effect on follow-up results, we would predict a difference between the two subsamples. If we failed to find one we could then exclude this unplanned event from our interpretation of the programme's effects. If we did find a difference between the 'CPN-visited' and the 'CPN-unvisited' clients we may still be able to salvage something useful from our study by distinguishing these two groups in our consideration of the results, as in estimating the incremental value of CPN visits over and above the programme effects.

More optimistically, unplanned changes may afford opportunities actually to improve the experiment. To offer a case in point, there was an outbreak of food poisoning in the sister hospital which led to the temporary closure of our day unit while the programme was being evaluated. Fortunately for research purposes, the closure interval very closely approximated to the evaluation interval, in which patients were assessed at the start and 3 months after starting attendance. Also, the initial assessments of a suitably large sample of patients had occurred immediately prior to the closure. In experimental terms this gave rise to a 'reversal' or control condition, allowing us to evaluate the effects of day hospital attendance against the effects of non-attendance for a similar group of clients.

Weiss (1972) suggests some other strategies for coping with unplanned changes, such as repeating earlier programme phases once unplanned changes have occurred. The results of both phases can then be compared, allowing us to judge the contribution made by any such changes. But, like Fairweather (1967), she also urges evaluators to try and anticipate such problems by obtaining as much control and consistency as possible over limited assessment and intervention periods. Tharp and Gallimore (1975) have provided a useful description of a further option, the 'developmental' strategy. In this approach any unplanned changes are incorporated into the analysis at a descriptive level as they arise, then are included systematically in subsequent evaluations. The notion behind this strategy is that programmes evolve in an organic way, making unplanned changes a natural corollary. They are therefore to be considered alongside the more deliberate changes that are introduced in successive programmes. The result is that we gradually exclude alternative explanations while simultaneously developing a more efficient programme. Jones (1979) has argued in a similar vein for the flexible use of different research designs. All these strategies represent possible solutions to the problems of standardising programmes. However, in the final analysis we may like to console ourselves with Campbell's (1969) wisdom on the problems of incidental change. Having done all we can to exert control over threats to the internal validity of our experiment, we can also take comfort that 'the mere possibility of an alternative explanation is not enough — it is only *plausible* rival hypotheses that are invalidating' (p. 411).

To conclude, let us consider the other main problem raised above, that of the inadequate description of a programme. Two solutions come to mind which may reduce this difficulty. The first is to minimise inconsistencies by ensuring that accurate records of what actually occurs are maintained. This could be achieved by a diary method, completed by the staff involved in each element of a programme. A more objective method would be to observe directly what is taking place at different times, in relation to the published programme. A time-sampling approach could be used during the evaluation period, so as to minimise effort and intrusion while maintaining scientific standards.

A clear illustration in objectively defining a programme has come from the Sheffield psychotherapy project. These researchers tape-recorded their interviews with patients and then classified the therapists' utterances during what were intended to be either 'exploratory' or 'prescriptive' phases of therapy. In this way they were able to show that what actually took place during these phases really did correspond with what should have happened, as defined by a manual (Hardy and Shapiro, 1985). They were thus able to demonstrate the 'integrity' of their therapy variable, and so could proceed confidently to interpret the results of each type of therapy.

An even more thorough approach to the description of programmes has been suggested by Schaffer (1982). He points out that many of our problems in teasing out the effects of different kinds of therapy are due to the very limited accounts we usually provide of our interventions. Three dimensions, he argues, need to be gauged if we are to offer a more useful description. They are measures of *what* was done (i.e. the kind of therapy — e.g. 'prescriptive' or 'exploratory'), of *how well* it was done (i.e. a skill or proficiency dimension), and of the interpersonal manner of the therapist. Moreover, it is suggested that each of these dimensions are assessed in different ways — for example, the 'type' of therapy is determined through audio-tape transcripts and blind codings (as in Hardy and Shapiro, 1985)

34

and that interpersonal manner is determined by the judgements of the clients. Table 2.3 presents the data derived from just such an evaluation, with an additional scale for 'clinical effectiveness' (Milne and Castle, 1986). It can be seen that the therapy provided in this study was behavioural in nature, was carried out with a 'satisfactory' degree of proficiency, that the patients regarded the therapist as high on interpersonal manner, and that 'experts' regarded it as 'effective' therapy.

2.5. MEASURING THE AMOUNT OF CHANGE THAT OCCURS

(a) Possible problems

There are two main difficulties in measuring change. One concerns the research design and is the subject of the next

Table 2.3: A detailed description of therapy

Evaluation dimensions	Measures applied	Evaluations made by	Results
'Type' of therapy	Helper Behaviour Rating Scale (Shapiro, Barkham and Irving, 1984) and 'experts' judgements	Two research assistants	'Behaviour therapy' (not e.g. 'cognitive therapy')
'Skill' or proficiency with which therapy conducted	Bi-polar rating scale, ranging from 0 ('poor') to 6 ('excellent') (Milne, 1986a)	Seven 'expert' clinicians	'Satisfactory' level of proficiency (3)
'Interpersonal manner'	Bi-polar scale ranging from 0 ('very low') to 6 ('very high'). Consumer Satisfaction Form (Milne, 1986c)	All patients included in the study and seven 'experts' using Cognitive Therapy Scale items (Young and Beck, 1980)	High endorsement for interpersonal manner (patients 5.3; 'experts' 4.4)
'Clinical effectiveness'	Bi-polar rating scale ranging from 0 ('in-effective') to 6 ('extremely effective') (Milne, 1986b)	Seven 'expert' clinicians	'Effective' (3.2)

section. The second involves the selection, adequacy and application of the measuring instruments or procedures that contribute to the design.

Many practitioners may not have ready access to suitable measures or to the libraries that may house them. Further, they may not have the training or experience to develop their own alternatives. An equally problematic situation can arise when measures are readily available but are inappropriate. Here again the practitioners' training may fail them. They may not know how to select the most appropriate measure from amongst those available. Considerations such as those concerning an instrument's reliability, validity or sensitivity may pass the practitioner by or get lost behind a barrage of more pressing issues. Forefront amongst these are problems in implementing a measurement procedure. This entails obstacles in the specific sense of introducing extra demands on staff or clients, and then problems in scheduling these into the programme. More generally it represents a change in the system; no simple matter and one that often elicits resistance (Liberman, 1979). Thus one may have the most appropriate measuring device available but be prevented from measuring changes in the client's condition due to practical constraints such as staff resistance to observation. For instance, researchers have reported that staff have defocused their video cameras so that they would not record nurse–patient interactions (Watson, 1979).

(b) Possible solutions

One obvious if impractical way of minimising problems in selecting measures is to receive specialised training. Baskin, Leversque, Macpherson *et al.* (1980), for instance, described a 'seminar programme' held in eight Canadian provinces for 300 health care participants. During the seminar they had the opportunity to discuss a research project of their own choosing with a tutor. The authors also developed a manual covering methods of health care evaluation, which had been distributed to almost 2,000 health service personnel. They reported satisfactory results from their training efforts in terms of facilitating research, and also provided a model for other countries to copy.

Other options include the various textbooks and local courses that are available on research methods, and another valuable resource can be an interest group or an individual with a specialised training in research methods, such as a psychologist. Finally, perhaps the most effective option is to learn research skills gradually, through one's own efforts. This has the advantage of making basic problems highly relevant to our own work experience, thus maintaining interest while we try out other solutions and so develop the necessary skills.

A solution to the selection problem is to employ several concurrent measures. This allows us to judge the relative value of different instruments or procedures in terms of our programme. Those that are difficult to apply or produce unreliable or invalid results can then be discarded in favour of the more sensitive and dependable measures. Barlow, Hayes and Nelson (1984) elaborate on these issues and Nelson (1981) has written a most helpful article in which she discusses the use of multiple measures, as well as describing some of the main ways of gathering clinical data. They include the methods of self-monitoring, self-ratings, card sorts, questionnaires, direct observation and physiological measures. She also gave consideration to the adequacy of these different indices for different problems.

Spevack and Gilman (1980) have generated an even longer list of possible measures, for use in behaviour therapy. They enumerate 26 different clinical problems and suggest ways of quantifying each of them objectively, ranging from the frequency of compulsive rituals to the percentage incapacity in writing with writer's cramp. Standard questionnaires were also listed, such as Beck's Depression Inventory (Beck, Ward, Mendelson et al., 1961). To these could be added a long list of carefully developed and readily applicable measures. Table 2.4 provides a small sample of these.

Should self-report questionnaires present difficulties in implementing an evaluation (for example, because the clients are unable to complete them by reason of their clinical problem) then the major alternative is direct observation or ratings made by staff. Some of the available measures are presented in Table 2.4. To offer a more detailed example, in our day hospital evaluations we adapted a structured interview (Platt, Weyman, Hirsch and Hewett, 1980) so that nurses could make systematic observations of individual clients. We christened this instrument the Behaviour Assessment Rating Scale (BARS), agreed on the meanings of terms it emphasised and ensured that nurses used it

Table 2.4: Some readily available clinical measures

Type of measure	Examples	Measures	Source
Questionnaire	Mobility inventory for agoraphobia	Agoraphobic avoidance and frequency of panic attacks	Chambless, Canputo, Jasin et al. (1985)
	Depression inventory	Depression	Beck et al. (1961)
	Coping responses questionnaire	Cognitive behavioural and affective ways of coping	Billings and Moos (1981)
	Self-efficacy scale	General and social effectiveness	Sherer, Maddax, Mercandante et al. (1982)
	Dyadic adjustment scale	Quality of marriage and similar dyads	Spanier (1976)
Structured interview	Social behaviour assessment schedule	Burden on relatives	Platt et al. (1980)
	Present state examination	Measurement and classification of psychiatric symptoms	Wing, Cooper and Sartorius (1974)
	Symptom rating scale	Rating of four aspects of chronic schizophrenia	Wing (1961)
Observation	Inpatient scale of minimal functioning	Low-level behaviour amongst chronic populations	Paul, Redfield and Lentz (1976)
	Behaviour observation instrument	Client activities in programmes	Alevizos, Derisi, Liberman et al. (1978)
	Attendant behaviour checklist	Nurses' behaviour on ward	Gardner and Giampa (1971)
	Nurses' observation scale for inpatient evaluation	Higher levels of functioning amongst chronic population	Honigfeld (1966)
	Staff–resident interaction chronograph	Nature, frequency and content of staff–client interactions	Paul and Lentz (1977)

in a reliable manner, by assessing inter-rater reliability (Milne, 1984). Ratings were practised until a satisfactorily high level of agreement was achieved, then observational evaluations could start. Table 2.5 lists some of the BARS categories and their definitions. Nurses rated each patient's behaviour in terms of 22 such categories, using a five-point scale, ranging from a frequency of 'very marked' to 'not at all'.

The results from the BARS were used to determine individual clinical change, but they could also be used to define the general range and degree of problems in a sample of clients, so facilitating programme planning.

The major alternative to using published measures in the kind of group design we have generally been describing is to utilise 'single-case' designs (Hersen and Barlow, 1976). In this experimental strategy each client is treated as his or her own control. After an initial baseline assessment of the frequency of a given problem, usually over a period of several days, various treatment elements are carefully introduced one at a time.

Figure 2.2, for example, is a summary of the effects of a

Table 2.5: Some of the categories and definitions of the BARS direct observation measure

Category	Definition
Withdrawal	Keeping to self, not approaching others or responding much if approached. Refusing or unwilling to participate in activities.
Odd ideas	Expressing unusual thoughts; may say something obviously untrue and usually bizarre.
Overactivity	Excessively cheerful, active, talkative, agitated, restless, unable to complete one thing at a time. Changing topic frequently, talking and moving rapidly and ceaselessly.
Irritability	Picking on people for little reason, easily upset, short-tempered, little tolerance, quick mood change, 'snappy' and bad-tempered.
Violence	Threatening, either verbally or physically towards anyone. Breaking or throwing things, pushing or hitting people, swearing or name-calling.
Hypochondria	Complains about bodily aches and pains, looking for sympathy and/or attention. 'Always' tired or ill or dissatisfied with service at hospital.

Figure 2.2: An illustrative summary from a single-case research design

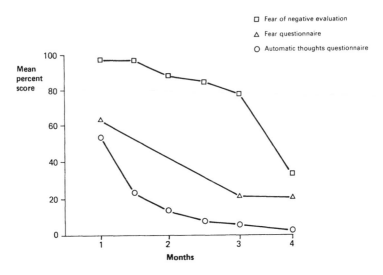

'package' of cognitive–behavioural treatment methods applied with a dysmorphobic client attending our illustrative day hospital. A baseline assessment of the problem included three questionnaires, the Fear Questionnaire (Marks and Matthews, 1979), Fear of Negative Evaluation (Watson and Friend, 1969) and the Automatic Thoughts Questionnaire (Hollon and Kendall, 1980). These were then re-administered throughout a 4-month period of day hospital attendance. The results indicate a major reduction in the patient's anxiety about her facial appearance by the end of this period, and this was supported by observations of increased social activities. The most severe problem at the baseline assessment, namely her extreme fear of being judged by others as abnormal, changed most dramatically between months 3 and 4. This was the point in time when we introduced an additional treatment approach, so we could infer that this was probably responsible for her improvement. Routine attendance at the day hospital, in contrast, seemed to have helped to reduce her general levels of social avoidance and depressed thoughts.

In addition to letting us know how much each element contributes to client improvement, the single-case design also has the considerable advantage of allowing us to determine individual variability in response to treatment. This information can often tell us much more than the results from group designs, because summaries of group outcomes may conceal large variations in the clients' response to treatment. Intensive study of such individual variability may well repay us more handsomely than group designs.

Single-case designs also favour the evaluation of change in terms of obvious clinical changes, rather than by determining their statistical significance. It is argued that the kinds of changes that are meaningful to practitioners are sufficiently definite not to require any statistical inference. Barlow *et al.* (1984), who present a strong argument for single-case research, provide the example of a group of anxious clients who all improved by 5 per cent. Although this would be statistically significant, it would not be clinically significant: neither clients nor therapist might notice the change. Barlow *et al.* (1984) argue that the traditional preoccupation with group designs and statistical significance have prevented the integration of scientists and practitioners. In contrast, single-case research, they believe, provides a bridge between the two camps and a ready introduction to research for the practitioner.

In more general terms, single-case designs are one relatively straightforward way of addressing the problems of execution, interpretation and replication raised above. They do not depend on published instruments, but are usually based on simple measures of the frequency, duration or intensity of a problem, easing both execution and interpretation. Also, by repeating the therapy, either with the same individual at different points in time or with successive clients, we can establish the generality of our results. This helps us to answer the long-standing question of which treatments, administered by which therapists, work best with which clients.

2.6 DETERMINING THE EXTENT TO WHICH CHANGE IS ATTRIBUTABLE TO THE PROGRAMME

(a) Possible problems

The essential problem facing the practitioner–scientist is that of teasing out the effects of a programme from the effects of other factors affecting the client's well-being. This is a classical research problem; one that experimental designs were intended to overcome. An experiment basically attempts to hold other factors constant while varying the one of interest in a systematic way and measuring its effect alone. While this is a relatively straightforward matter in the laboratory, it is an unattainable ideal in the mental health services.

In the face of such difficulty the practitioner may be tempted to abandon the attempt at being scientific. But here again it may be that their training and experience are at fault, rather than there being any insurmountable obstacles in their research plans and setting. This is not to minimise the very considerable difficulties facing all evaluative researchers in interpreting any findings they may derive from a study. Given that truly rigorous experimental designs are not viable in health services settings, then we are usually left to infer the effects of a programme in a very cautious manner. It is all too possible that an effect we have attributed to our programme is really due to something we didn't or couldn't measure.

(b) Possible solutions

It is not essential to have other variables constant while determining the effect of a programme, although this is, of course, a highly desirable state of affairs. For one thing, some changes may assist the evaluation process, as in the example cited earlier when food poisoning closed our day hospital and created a natural control group. Provided regular measures are taken of the programme's effects, then the results of unplanned changes can be assessed separately.

To illustrate, in our 'ward atmosphere' evaluation of the day hospital we measured the nurses' perceptions before making any changes in the programme. We assessed these a second time after the clients had been divided into two groups ('acute' and 'chronic') so as to gauge the effect of this change alone. Then we conducted a third assessment of their perceptions, having introduced the programme changes. This allowed us to be fairly confident that the grouping had not affected the ward atmosphere, whereas programme changes had. If we had not taken our measurements between these two changes we would not be able to say which of them was responsible for the improved ward atmosphere.

Kraemer (1981) has written a refreshingly frank account of such problems in research design. She has indicated a number of ways in which we might cope with unplanned changes and how we might manage to start studies under routine (i.e. difficult) clinical conditions. The sample size, for instance, need not necessarily be more than twenty in a group research design, with ten in a treated group and ten assigned to control conditions. Subjects do not have to be randomly selected for these groups, since a convenient sample can still be described systematically, so that we can subsequently decide which population they represent. She offers equally encouraging advice with regard to randomly assigning clients to treatment groups, and with the design and analysis of the study. This leads her to advocate a critical but inventive approach to research, one that encourages us to conduct the best possible evaluation. In turn, this increases our confidence in judging the extent to which the programme was responsible for the obtained results.

2.7 ASSESSING THE RELATIVE EFFECTIVENESS OF MODIFIED PROGRAMMES

(a) Possible problems

This final feature of evaluative research concerns its educational potential. Ideally, we not only want to know the extent to which a programme achieved its goals, but also how we might improve it next time around. The term 'formative' evaluation has been used to refer to this function (Scriven, 1972).

Some of the problems in this sphere follow directly from the issues already raised about the experience of practitioners. For example, as we learn more about how best to measure client change, we tend to change the measures: we decide that we need 'better' ways of evaluating their response to therapy. This may enhance the next evaluation, but it simultaneously reduces our capacity to relate a series of programme changes to one another, since we are comparing different programmes using different measures, so creating problems of interpretation.

In a similar way the growing experience of the practitioner-scientist may dictate 'better' experimental designs. These are equally capable of annulling comparisons over time. The very fact that an earlier evaluation has taken place may also encourage colleagues to become interested, adding the changes they may wish to introduce to the experimental design. Also, with experience the practitioner tends to move on to other service positions or to different problems. The funding or support that may be available for an initial project are not typically made available for the evaluation of subsequent modifications in a programme. Baer (1981) wryly notes that first evaluations are much more likely to be funded, even though subsequent programmes are likely to be more effective. He suggests that this is partly due to the fact that such derived programmes are seen as 'boring'. However, although the first programme is more likely to excite, it is the derivatives that contribute most to our understanding and control.

(b) Possible solutions

The most straightforward way of dealing with changes in the measurement of programmes is to try and retain at least one measure as a reference point. This is particularly valuable when there is an outcome that everyone accepts as essential, such as discharge from a rehabilitation ward. Such a measure can serve as a criterion against which other measures may be judged. For instance, if a new social skills test predicts successful discharge better than one that was used in earlier evaluations, we would prefer it. We would also be interested in refining measures so that they are economical to apply, as in self-report assessments such as the General Health Questionnaire (GHQ; Goldberg, 1978) which can save interview time without great losses in accuracy.

Changes in the overall research design can also make evaluation more efficient. Suchman (1970), for instance, points out that not all evaluative studies require the same degree of scientific rigour, and that many administrative decisions can be made on the basis of limited evaluations. He suggested that future studies should develop our understanding of the different forms an evaluation can take and when each is adequate and appropriate.

In keeping with our emphasis on a gradual 'learning' approach to the acquisition of evaluative research skills, Suchman (1970) has also proposed a four-stage 'developmental' process. This distinguishes a 'pilot' phase, involving early trial-and-error experimentation, from a 'model' phase, when more control is introduced. The subsequent phases are the 'prototype' phase, in which the model programme is subjected to realistic working conditions; and finally an 'institutionalised' phase during which the new programme becomes integrated into the everyday workings of the unit. He argues that it is only in the model phase that the programme must be held stable for experimental investigation. At the other phases less systematic control is required and unplanned changes are to be expected and tolerated.

In short, an inventive and flexible approach to experimental methods can generate solutions to most of the problems that arise in service settings. It should be noted that this is not the same as commending sloppy research. Parker and Thomas (1980) are quite correct to mock the 'fads, flaws, fallacies and foolishness' of evaluative research, in which the belief that 'something is better that nothing' stands out as an all-too-common standard, leading to very rudimentary measurement and in turn to ill-conceived decisions about programmes. Campbell (1969) regards such poor experimental standards as leading into 'a morass of obfuscation and self-deception' (p. 426).

Rather, we are advocating that researchers seek the highest possible standards of experimental rigour. The limits that circumstances place on a study should be the main constraint, not the minimal standards often accepted by institutions or journals. Given a willingness to learn about research, these constraints can be considerably reduced and valuable, 'tight' studies can emerge. This seems to be particularly likely in successive evaluations of a programme, since practitioners can learn to do steadily better research.

2.8   SUMMARY AND CONCLUSIONS

In this chapter we have used the characteristic features of evaluative research as a framework for discussing possible problems and solutions in conducting evaluations. A psychiatric day hospital provided illustrations and an attempt was made to be realistic but constructive. There are undoubtedly many major obstacles to overcome in studying service settings systematically, but there are an almost equally large range of solutions available.

In discussing the problems in setting programme goals, for instance, we suggested the use of the Ward Atmosphere Scale and similar instruments. Another compatible strategy is to conduct a problem census of clients who are served by a programme. This can also help to define the service tasks we need to undertake. A recurring point was how a flexible and imaginative use of research designs and measures could minimise problems in judging the extent to which the programme produced the outcomes we achieved. A 'developmental' perspective was suggested, in which the sophistication of our research efforts progressed in terms of the kinds of questions we were addressing and our own level of competence. Gradually we could learn, through the experience of conducting progressively more exacting studies, how to do better research on more difficult issues. This 'self-help' approach underlined our practitioner–scientist philosophy, although we recognised the value of formal training or of more experienced colleagues as guides that might well facilitate learning.

In a comparable sense, we could imagine how our programmes might also 'learn' through repeated evaluation. If each analysis serves to reduce the useless elements and increase the valuable ones our service can change in an orderly way, yielding better results along the way. As well as benefiting the clients who use the programme it may also help the practitioners who operate it, since evaluation data can serve to let them know how to develop their skills and give them an objective sense of effectiveness, which usually helps motivation and morale.

ACKNOWLEDGEMENTS

I am indebted to the staff and patients of Stanley Royd Day Hospital for their involvement and support throughout this evaluation, especially Margaret Stephenson, Cath Heaslip, Tim Burton, Chris Bontoft and Jane Throssall.

REFERENCES

Alevizos, P., Derisi, W., Liberman, R., Eckman, T. and Callahan, E. (1978) 'The Behavior Observation Instrument: A Method for Direct Observation for Programme Evaluation', *Journal of Applied*

Behavior Analysis, 11, 243-57

Baer, D.M. (1981) 'The Nature of Intervention Research'. In: *Early Language: Acquisition and Intervention,* University Park Press, Baltimore, Md

Barlow, D.H., Hayes, S.C. and Nelson, R.O. (1984) *The Scientist–Practitioner,* Pergamon Press, New York.

Baskin, M., Levesque, L., Macpherson, A.S., Poole, P.E. and Sackett, D.L. (1980) 'Canada's Health Care Evaluation Seminars: An Epilogue and Evaluation', *Canadian Journal of Public Health, 71,* 321-7

Beck, A.T., Ward, C.H., Mendelson, M., Mock, J. and Erbaugh, J. (1961) 'An Inventory for Measuring Depression', *Archives of General Psychiatry, 4,* 53-63

Billings, A.G. and Moos, R.H. (1981) 'The Role of Coping Responses and Social Resources in Attenuating the Stress of Life Events', *Journal of Behavioural Medicine, 4,* 139-57

Campbell, D.T. (1969) 'Reforms as Experiments', *American Psychologist, 24,* 409-29

Campbell, D.T. and Stanley, J.C. (1963) *Experimental and Quasi-Experimental Designs for Research,* Rand McNally, Chicago, Ill.

Chambless, D.L., Canputo, G.C., Jasin, S.E., Gracely, E.J. and Williams, C. (1985) 'The Mobility Inventory for Agoraphobia', *Behaviour Research and Therapy, 23,* 35-44

Cochrane, A.L. (1972) *Effectiveness and Efficiency,* Nuffield Provincial Hospitals Trust, London

Fairweather, G.W. (1967) *Methods for Experimental Social Innovation,* Wiley, New York

Freeman, H.E. and Sherwood, C.C. (1965) 'Research in Large Scale Intervention Programmes', *Journal of Social Issues, 21,* 11-28

Gardner, J.M. and Giampa, F.L. (1971) 'The Attendant Behavior Checklist: Measuring on the Ward Behavior of Institutional Attendants', *American Journal of Mental Deficiency, 75,* 617-22

Goldberg, D. (1978) *Manual of the General Health Questionnaire,* NFER, Windsor

Hardy, G.E. and Shapiro, D.A. (1985) 'Therapist Response Modes in Prescriptive vs. Exploratory Psychotherapy', *British Journal of Clinical Psychology, 24,* 235-45

Hersen, M. and Barlow, D.H. (1976) *Single Case Experimental Designs: Strategies for Studying Behavior Change,* Pergamon, New York

Hollon, S.D. and Kendall, P.C. (1980) 'Cognitive Self-statements in Depression: Development of an Automatic Thoughts Questionnaire', *Cognitive Therapy and Research, 4,* 383-95

Honigfeld, G. (1966) *Nurses' Observation Scale for In-Patient Evaluation (NOSIE-30),* Honigfeld: Glen Oakes, New York

Jones, R.R. (1979) 'Programme Evaluation Design Issues', *Behavioural Assessment, 1,* 51-6

Kraemer, H.C. (1981) 'Coping Strategies in Psychiatric Clinical Research', *Journal of Consulting and Clinical Psychology, 49,* 309-19

Liberman, R.P. (1979) 'Social and Political Challenges to the Development of Behavioural Programmes in Organizations', in: P. Sjoden, S. Bates and W.S. Dockens III (eds), *Trends in Behavior Therapy*, Academic Press, New York

Lloyd, M.E. (1983) 'Selecting Systems to Measure Client Outcome in Human Service Agencies', *Behavioural Assessment*, 5, 55-70

Marks, I.M. and Mathews, A.M. (1979) 'Brief Standard Self-rating for Phobic Patients', *Behaviour Research and Therapy*, 17, 263-7

Milne, D.L. (1984) 'A Comparative Evaluation of Two Psychiatric Day Hospitals', *British Journal of Psychiatry*, 145, 533-7

Milne, D.L. (1986a) 'Planning and Evaluating Innovations in Nursing Practice by Measuring the Ward Atmosphere', *Journal of Advanced Nursing*, 11, 203-10

Milne, D.L. (1986b) 'Organisational Behaviour Management in a Psychiatric Day Hospital' *Behavioural Psychotherapy* (in press)

Milne, D.L. and Castle, F. (1986) 'A Process Evaluation of a Routine Clinical Psychology Service'. Paper presented at the annual conference of the British Association for Behavioural Psychotherapy, Manchester

Milne, D.L. and Mullin, M. (1987) 'Is a Problem Shared a Problem Shaved? An empirical analysis of informal psychotherapy'. *British Journal of Clinical Psychology*, 26, 69-70

Moss, R.H. (1974) *Evaluating Treatment Environments: A Social-Ecological Approach*, Wiley, London

Nelson, R.O. (1981) 'Realistic Dependent Measures for Clinical Use', *Journal of Consulting and Clinical Psychology*, 49, 168-82

Parker, R.M. and Thomas, K.R. (1980) 'Fads, Flaws, Fallacies and Foolishness in Evaluation of Rehabilitation Programmes', *Journal of Rehabilitation*, 46, 32-4

Paul, G.L. and Lentz, R.J. (1977) *Psychosocial Treatment of Chronic Mental Patients: Milieu Versus Social Learning Programmes*, Harvard University Press, Cambridge, Mass.

Paul, G.L., Redfield, J.P. and Lentz, R.J. (1976) 'The In-patient Scale of Minimal Functioning: a Revision of the Social Breakdown Syndrome Gradient Index', *Journal of Consulting and Clinical Psychology*, 44, 1021-2

Peterson, L., Homer, A.L. and Wonderlich, S.A. (1982) 'The Integrity of Independent Variables in Behaviour Analysis', *Journal of Applied Behavior Analysis*, 15, 477-92

Platt, S., Weyman, A., Hirsch, S. and Hewett, S. (1980) 'The Social Behaviour Assessment Schedule (SBAS): Rationale, Contents, Scoring and Reliability of a New Interview Schedule', *Social Psychiatry*, 15, 43-55

Schaffer, N.D. (1982) 'Multidimensional Measures of Therapist Behaviour as Predictors of Outcome', *Psychological Bulletin*, 92, 670-81

Scriven, M. (1972) 'The Methodology of Evaluation'. In: C.H. Weiss (ed.), *Evaluating Action Programmes*, Allyn & Bacon, Boston, Massachusetts

Shapiro, D.A. Barkham, M. and Irving, D.L. (1980) 'A Modified Helper Behaviour Rating System'. University of Sheffield SAPU

Memo 415.

Sherer, M., Maddux, J.E., Mercandante, B., Prentice-Dunn, S., Jacobs, B., and Rogers, R.W. (1982) 'The Self-efficacy Scale: Construction and Validation', *Psychological Reports, 51,* 663-71

Spanier, G.B. (1976) 'Measuring Dyadic Adjustment: New Scales for Assessing the Quality of Marriage and Similar Dyads', *Journal of Marriage and The Family,* February, pp. 15-27

Spevack, M. and Gilman, S. (1980) 'A System for Evaluative Research in Behaviour Therapy', *Psychotherapy: Theory, Research and Practice, 17,* 37-43

Stanley, B. (1984) 'Evaluation of Treatment Goals: the Use of Goal Attainment Scaling', *Journal of Advanced Nursing, 9,* 351-6

Suchman, E.A. (1970) 'Action for What? A Critique of Evaluative Research'. In: R. O'Tool (ed.), *The Organization, Management and Tactics of Social Research,* Schenkman, Cambridge, Mass.

Tharp, R.G. and Gallimore, R. (1975) 'The Ecology of Programme Research and Evaluation'. In: L. Sechrest, S.G. West, M.A. Philips, R. Redner and W. Yeaton (eds) *Evaluation Studies Review Manual,* vol. 4, Sage, Beverley Hills, Calif.

Watson, D. and Friend, R. (1969) 'Measurement of Social–Evaluative Anxiety', *Journal of Consulting and Clinical Psychology, 33,* 448-57

Watson, W.H. (1979) 'Resistances to Naturalistic Observation in a Geriatric Setting'. *International Journal of Aging and Human Development, 10,* 35-45

Weiss, C.H. (1972) *Evaluation Research,* Prentice-Hall, Englewood-Cliffs, NJ

Winefield, H.R. (1984) 'The Nature and Elicitation of Social Support: Some Implications for the Helping Professions', *Behavioural Psychotherapy, 12,* 318-30

Wing, J.K., (1961) 'A Simple and Reliable Subclassification of Chronic Schizophrenia', *Journal of Mental Science, 107,* 862-75

Wing, J.K. Cooper, J.E. and Sartorius, N. (1974) *Measurement and Classification of Psychiatric Symptoms,* Cambridge University Press, Cambridge

Young, J.E. and Beck, A.T. (1980) 'Cognitive Therapy Scale Rating Manual', Center for Cognitive Therapy, University of Pennsylvania, Room 602, 133 S. 36th Street, Philadelphia, PA 19104, USA

Part Two:
Reviews and Illustrations

3

Evaluation in Art Therapy

David Edwards

EDITOR'S INTRODUCTION

Our first chapter devoted to a specific mental health discipline provides an overview of evaluation in art therapy. Although the alphabetical order of disciplines adopted in the book dictated that art therapy should appear first, it is in any case a very suitable starting point. This is so because art therapy represents a clear illustration of some of the issues that surface in an emerging discipline, particularly when it is faced with increasing pressure to provide objective evidence of its utility. David Edwards highlights the doubt and confusion concerning the therapy's aims, methods and effectiveness in a way that may appear remarkably familiar to members of other disciplines! Moreover, he draws attention to the sporadic and unsystematic involvement of art therapists in evaluative reseach to date, the trend for therapists to accept responsibility for evaluating their work in the future, and the difficulties this introduces. All of these observations should be recognisable to fellow mental health disciplines.

Not least, this chapter is a helpful starting point in that it exemplifies the book's constructive emphasis. Having addressed the difficulties, David Edwards goes on to discuss ways in which a balance can be struck between objective methods of enquiry and a subjectively based therapy. He concludes by pointing to the potential benefits of the 'single-subject' approach to evaluation, as in developing our understanding of the most potent change processors in art therapy, and provides his own examples of how to enter into service evaluation.

3.1. INTRODUCTION

In Britain and North America art therapy is a relatively recent addition to the range of psychotherapies available through the mental health services, with the term itself generally acknowledged to have been first introduced in the USA during the 1940s by Margaret Naumberg. Although the status of the profession differs in a number of respects in North America and elsewhere, in Britain art therapy is now recognised as a postgraduate profession and no-one may be employed as an art therapist in the National Health Service without first having successfully completed one of the three training courses currently approved by the Department of Health and Social Security.

Art therapists may now be found working in a number of different areas of the mental health services; including psychiatric hospitals and units, mental handicap hospitals, in social service establishments and prisons. Within these broad areas art therapists may work with individuals on a one-to-one basis or with groups. Increasingly they are also to be found practising in a number of specialised fields such as family therapy, with the elderly and in community settings. In her survey of art therapists working in Britain, Liebmann (1981, pp. 26-8) observes that 'These very different working situations seemed to be a major influence on art therapists' methods of working.' Leibmann notes too that the purpose of art therapy may also vary according to the client group, ranging from encouraging personal autonomy and motivation to working with fantasy and the unconscious.

Although art therapy has, as Waller states, 'developed considerably from its informal and ill-defined beginning', and that 'supported by their specialist training, art therapists feel more confident in taking on the role of primary therapist and in effecting change where possible and desirable' (Waller, 1984, p. 14), this rapid development of an emergent profession has undoubtedly left in its wake a legacy of doubt and confusion concerning its aims and methods. That is with respect to both the theoretical assumptions upon which the practice of art therapy is based, and the value of that practice to clients or patients.

The confusing picture presented by art therapy, particularly to those unconvinced by its effectiveness, is one to which art therapists themselves have contributed, coming as they do from 'varying backgrounds and having different ways of working and describing what they do' (Rubin, 1982, p. 57). This situation is further complicated by the fact that practitioners from a variety of backgrounds in the mental health professions either use images directly in their work, or claim a degree of expertise in their therapeutic application. Commenting on the various approaches to the image when using art in therapy, including those taken by art therapists themselves, Watkins notes that there exists no natural kinship between therapists who depend upon images for their theories or therapeutic technique; adding 'Nor does the founding of a single kind of therapy (for instance art and therapy or sand play therapy) coalesce its group of practitioners. Within it there will be radical differences in approach to the imaginal' (Watkins, 1981, p. 107). These radical differences in approach are as evident in the means employed to evaluate art therapy as they are in the practice of art therapy itself.

In part, the existence of such differences in approach may be found rooted in those disciplines and theoretical constructs which have largely informed and influenced the development of art therapy to date. Pre-eminent amongst these are ideas drawn from psychoanalysis and psychotherapy, aesthetics, philosophy, education and psychiatry. To speak, therefore, of art therapy as though it were a systematised body of knowledge subscribed to by all those who would employ the use of images in treatment settings, or to convey the impression that art therapists are primarily concerned with the use of standardised techniques in the treatment of particular problems or client groups, would be to present a distorted view of a complex and developing field. In practice art therapy remains a young profession actively engaged in the difficult process of defining its own boundaries.

Mindful of the fact that art therapy is a term often used to describe a range of practices encompassing aspects of psycho-therapy, education and much in between, numerous definitions have been advanced with the aim of limiting the scope of its use. Rubin, for example, states that 'The essence of art therapy is that it must partake of both parts of its name — it must involve art and therapy. The goal of the art activity, therefore, must be primarily therapeutic' (Rubin, 1982, p. 57). This view of art therapy is echoed by Ulman, who regards its aims as being directed towards assisting 'favourable changes in personality or in living that will outlast the session itself' (Ulman, 1961, p. 19).

This definition is offered by Ulman to distinguish the aims of art therapy 'from those activities designed to offer only distraction from inner conflicts; activities whose benefits are, therefore, at best momentary' (Ulman, 1961, p. 19). While most art therapists would now accept such a definition of art therapy, what constitutes favourable change often varies according to the theoretical or philosophical perspective of the therapist, and the needs and resources of those involved in the therapeutic process. Thus, as Waller states, 'the goals of art therapy depend on the individuals with whom one works and these goals may change as the therapeutic relationship develops. For one patient, it may mean encouraging them to drop their verbal defences and get in touch with some feelings; for others to enable them to hold a crayon and make a mark' (Waller, 1984, p. 14). Similarly Holtom, in his 1976 survey of art therapists working in hospital settings, reports art therapists attributing an equally wide range of change in patients as the outcome of their interventions; including 'less frustration, inhibition, and more independence, concentration, openness and awareness' (Holtom, 1977, p. 34).

Although Holtom's survey of practising art therapists gives no indication as to the means employed by them when evaluating the nature and extent of the change observed in individuals, a unique feature of art therapy is that the permanence of the artwork produced during the process of therapy can be particularly useful in enabling both the therapist and client to follow and reflect upon changes which occur over a period of time. In addition to those benefits which may accrue through making images, the durability of the artwork itself has long provided the means by which the clinical application of art in therapy may be evaluated. However, by far the greater proportion of the published research in this area is concerned with the use of art as a means of diagnostic assessment as opposed to evaluating the process and outcome of art therapy.

3.2 ART AND PSYCHOPATHOLOGY

Interest in the artwork produced by psychiatric patients in particular pre-dates the emergence of art therapy by a considerable period of time, having been discussed and studied from three main perspectives: the psychiatric, the psychoanalytic and the artistic. Commenting upon the development of these studies in their review of the literature Anastasi and Foley (1944, p. 169) note: 'Relatively little of a conclusive nature can, however, be gleaned from the voluminous literature in this field, owing to the inadequate control of experimental conditions, and to the excessive theoretical speculation which frequently obscures the data.' Some subsequent investigations into the relationship between art and psychopathology have attempted to eliminate subjective bias from the process of clinical evaluation and diagnosis through employing more rigorously controlled methods of research; e.g. Anastasi and Foley (1944), Lehmann and Risquez (1953), Cunningham-Dax (1953), and Swenson (1968). The validity and outcome of this research nevertheless remains far from convincing or conclusive (Russell-Lacy, Robinson, Benson and Crange, 1979; Henzell, 1985).

Despite this uncertainty, research of this kind has exerted a marked influence on the development of art therapy, especially in North America, and in recent years art therapists themselves have begun to contribute increasingly to it. Gantt and Schmal (1974) in their comprehensive review of the relevant published literature between 1940 and 1973 list 87 references concerned with the use of art therapy in diagnosis and psychiatric evaluation; and a further 39 concerned with statistical studies in this area. Ulman (1965), Wadeson (1979) and Kwiatkowska (1978), for example, have developed standardised procedures in their work with individuals and families for eliciting and evaluating material under the controlled conditions believed to be useful in making diagnostic assessments. In these procedures emphasis is placed on the spontaneous nature of the material produced (in contrast to the procedures adopted in more orthodox psychological tests such as the Rorcharch 'ink-blot' test), and on the comments made about these images by their creator. Although subjectivity is acknowledged, as Kwiatkowska notes, 'methodical ways of obtaining and using patients' art for psychodynamic evaluation are necessary, in order to study material that can be systematically analysed and compared' (1973, p. 121). The necessity for art therapists working in North America to be able to make accurate diagnoses of psychiatric conditions from images, primarily as a means of gaining acceptance for and legitimising their practice, has prompted research in the field of training itself, with notably mixed results. Levy and Ulman, for example, have systematically evaluated the accuracy of art therapists as diagnosticians, basing their research on the belief that 'art therapists need to cultivate such a skill in order to make their work as effective as possible' (1974, p. 24).

3.3 EVALUATIVE RESEARCH IN ART THERAPY

In Britain this belief is not generally shared by practicing art therapists, or their medical colleagues. However, while art therapists have demonstrated little interest in statistically based evaluative research *through* art therapy, this also applies to research *in* art therapy; with such research as has been conducted having been 'sporadic and unsystematic' (Dalley, 1984, p. xxv). Commenting on the paucity of scientifically orientated research into art therapy Males has observed that 'in terms of objective research based on scientific measurement that can be put to general use, there sometimes appears to be an element of resistance amongst art therapists' (Males, 1979, p. 5). Such a view is borne out by a review of *Inscape*, the journal of the British Association of Art Therapists, over the period 1968 to 1985, which reveals only three papers referring directly to research issues and only one with scientific approaches to evaluating the efficacy of art therapy.

Developing her argument in a later paper Males states:

If art therapy is going to effect 'favourable changes' that are going to last then it surely is necessary to examine those changes in order to ensure that they are for the ultimate good. This is perhaps an ethical rather than academic issue: In this sense the right to treat an individual without knowledge of the efficacy of the treatment should be questioned. If art therapy is to be held in the esteem for which many would hope, it must stand up to investigation, examination, enquiry (Males, 1980, p. 13).

The method of enquiry preferred and developed by Males and her colleagues in their work with mentally handicapped adults adopted a behavioural approach basing its rationale upon procedures derived from orthodox scientific research methodology. The declared aim was to elicit 'objective statements of fact, rather than subjective description based on intuition'

(Males, 1980, p. 14). As this example of evaluative research in art therapy is a unique example of its kind, and as the researchers themselves argue that their work has implications for the development of art therapy outside the field of mental handicap, it merits detailed discussion.

The research project was conducted over a 2-year period as a co-operative venture between the art therapy and clinical psychology departments, and was aided by funding from the Department of Health and Social Security. It aimed at a systematic comparison between the two main methods of working commonly found to be used by art therapists practicing in mental handicap; that is, with directive approaches emphasising skill learning within a developmental structure, and non-directive approaches aimed at fostering and developing independence, choice and exploration. This was felt to be necessary because there was only limited evidence available regarding the relative usefulness of the two methods (Crawford, 1962). Fifty-seven subjects were involved in the research project, each of whom participated in one of six groups for a 26-week period. Non-art-based activities in occupational therapy acted as a control. The measures used were selected in order to obtain information from three main areas believed relevant to the application of art therapy in mental handicap; general behaviour in and out of sessions, social competence, and the artwork. Standard methods of measuring observed behaviour were used whenever possible, and a developmental assessment plan developed for studying the artwork. Once the data had been collated four major findings were revealed:

(1) That the means used to evaluate the artwork indicated little change over the period of assessment, possibly due to the categories of measurement being too broad to identify gradual change, or the actual change having been slight.

(2) In all three groups little differentiation was found in the overall general positive therapeutic effect; that is, in the maintenance of existing skills and improvements in 'appropriate' behaviour, defined as active, adaptive behaviour observed in the context of learning new skills. Although this was regarded as disappointing in one sense by the researchers, in as much as it did not clearly demonstrate the superiority of one approach or form of therapy compared to another, this finding was nevertheless regarded as helpful

in refuting the notion that art therapy is no more than a pleasing time-filler.

(3) Interesting data were revealed concerning the consistency of the therapists' ratings. Therapists were found to be most consistent in their views regarding the benefits gained by an individual from art therapy when their self-expression was well developed, they developed new ideas, concentrated on the task in therapy, and responded to the therapist. While a high level of consistency was found between the raters, statistical analysis of the assessments did not, however, reveal any significant change in the patients. One possible explanation for this was the infrequency of the ratings and the limited experimental period, which may have been too short to reveal any observable change in the patient group.

(4) By developing a new method of analysing the available data which relied less on average scores and more on the performance of individuals, interesting and useful information was revealed concerning the level of dependence and the degree of self-expression observed. For an individual to be seen as making progress in therapy the extent of self-expression was found to be the most significant factor for the most dependent individuals.

Summarising the foregoing research Stott concludes:

The difficulties in undertaking research in art therapy are often highlighted at the same time as the importance of research is underlined. The present study has shown that it is possible to use research methods from a speciality area without impinging excessively on the treatment, and at the same time produce data that will have practical consequences for clinicians (Stott, 1985, p. 5).

Although evaluative research in art therapy employing methods of enquiry derived from the physical and human sciences remains very much in its infancy, serious attempts have been made, as the previous example clearly illustrates, to demonstrate objectively the efficacy of art therapy. However, while those researchers employing such methods attach considerable importance to their findings, the profession as a whole remains largely uninfluenced by them. Similarly, Serban's critical study of the use of art therapy in treating psychotic patients has not deterred art therapists from working with this client group (Serban, 1972). The reluctance of practising art therapists to take seriously or engage in similar research may, as Holtom notes, 'be a result of a healthy unwillingness on the part of art therapists to subject their work to paramedical or pseudo-medical dissection' (Holtom, 1977, p. 36). It may also be that existing methodological approaches to the problems of research in art therapy are regarded as 'not necessarily sensitive to the special attributes of communication through art expression' (Wadeson, 1980, p. 318).

While most, if not all, art therapists would now accept that they have a responsibility to evaluate their work, the most appropriate means of doing so remains a moot point. It is certainly not the case that the 'reluctance' of practitioners to engage in research basing its methods on procedures derived from orthodox scientific enquiry may be explained simply as 'resistance', procrastination or indifference. To do so would be naive, and to ignore the impact which critics who were sceptical of the claims made on behalf of scientific objectivity, as applied to understanding and responding to human distress and need through psychological and psychiatric intervention, have had upon training in and the practice of art therapy. Thus Edwards, commenting upon the current state of research in art therapy is able to state:

> the realisation has grown that research is not necessarily best served by the laboratory model but rather by lines of serious enquiry which most appropriately reflect the essentials of the subject being investigated. Recent interest in phenomeno-logical approaches, when subjectivity is freely acknowledged as appropriate to certain forms of enquiry, indicate that old research models may be changing (Edwards, 1981, p. 21).

Lines of reasoning such as this have exerted considerable influence within art therapy, particularly within the area of training where the individual case study approach to research remains the most popular means of illustrating and evaluating the kinds of things which happen in the therapeutic situation. However, while the case study does acknowledge the uniqueness of the patient–therapist encounter and the special circumstances in which this encounter takes place, the reporting of events and the significance attached to these tends to be described solely from the perspective of the therapist.

For those critical of research in art therapy for emphasising subjective as opposed to objective evaluations of process and outcome, case studies or case histories are often regarded as idiosyncratic and untrustworthy; not because they necessarily lack the rigour of serious enquiry but through a failure to provide data of the kind necessary to attain the status of verifiable fact. For this reason practitioners and researchers in allied fields such as psychotherapy, where 'facts' remain at a premium and the discipline is one largely dominated by psychiatrists and clinical psychologists with 'scientific' backgrounds, have by and large stopped short of abandoning the methods of scientific enquiry entirely. Nevertheless, questions arising out of the issue of whether or not the complexities of understanding human conduct are best served by methods of enquiry derived from the natural sciences, and disillusion with the methodological problems involved when attempting to conduct controlled experiments in clinical settings, has led to a growth of interest in applied or evaluative research. That is, research which is more concerned with generating information about the process and outcome of therapy relevant to the needs of practitioners than with 'facts' *per se* (Hobson and Shapiro, 1970; Malan, 1973; Bergin and Lambert, 1978). Moreover, as practitioners are primarily concerned with individuals experiencing particular difficulties in particular settings, generalised research findings calculating the statistical significance of measures comparing one form of intervention with another, or none at all, tend to have little or no influence on their work. Far from providing a basis from which practitioners might better understand what is and what is not helpful about their interventions such research has, as Barlow *et al.* note, 'served to widen the scientist–practitioner gap' (Barlow, Hayes and Nelson, 1984, p. 32). Similarly, Yalom has observed 'Clinicians fail to heed or even believe research in which outcome is measured by before–after changes in the MMPI or some other standardised instrument, and with good reason, for there is abundant clinical and research evidence to indicate change means something different to each patient' (Yalom, 1974, p. 519). In practice, psychological therapists of all persuasions — including art therapists — are more likely to base their sense of efficacy upon the orientation of their training, the personal influence of colleagues, and their own clinical experience than upon research findings which often seem unhelpful or irrelevant.

Although the 'trial-and-error' experience of art therapists might not unreasonably be said to have contributed to the development of the profession, and benefited those in need through its expansion into new areas, the fact remains that such progress has relied less upon empirical research than the creative intuition and persuasive influence of individual practitioners. In part this situation may be explained as one finding its origin in the assumption that empirical research is essentially separate from and not, as may be the case, simply a more thorough-going form of, the trial-and-error experience of practitioners. It must also be acknowledged, however, that all research in art therapy, but particularly empirical research, has undoubtedly been hampered by such factors as the fear of criticism and failure, inexperience and lack of confidence in using available research skills, the lack of support for and interest in research, and ultimately the routine demands of the work itself. At the present time few art therapists are in a position to conduct large-scale evaluative research projects in art therapy; with those who are able to do so having to fund their research out of their own resources, under the auspices of postgraduate training programmes at MA, MPhil and PhD levels. Without a major change in attitude from employing authorities it is difficult to see how this situation might improve.

However, given the practical constraints upon the development of relatively complex research strategies, one possible way forward might be for art therapists to focus upon an individual analysis of their work paying particular attention to change, degree of change, lack of change and the reasons for any lack of change. Two early examples of the individual case study approach to evaluating the art therapy process systematically are provided by Dalley (1979, 1980), each combining an assessment of the patients' artwork together with the use of self-rating questionnaires. Although both studies might be said to have been weakened by the absence of any control to take account of the influence factors outside the art therapy sessions may have had upon the progress of therapy, the use of images when combined with the individual patients' own ratings along a range of dimensions (e.g. relaxed–anxious, involved–isolated, etc.) can, as Dalley argues, offer a 'detailed insight into the dynamics of the therapeutic process' (Dalley, 1980, p. 15), insights which might provide information not immediately apparent but none the less useful in assessing the short- or long-term development of therapy.

Ethically and practically the process of evaluating change attributable to art therapy would need to be consistent with a sensitive clinical approach, that is, one based in a personal relationship as mediated through the image; in addition to taking full account of the fact that what constitutes 'favourable' change may very well vary according to the views of the referring agent, therapist and patient.

In practice such an approach could involve systematically collecting data from referring agents and patients regarding the reasons for undertaking art therapy; assessing the severity of the problem before and after therapy according to the view of the referring agent and the patient; assessments by the patient and the therapist of change in the therapeutic relationship and imagery over a period of time through observation and self-assessments; and post-therapy assessment of outcome by the referring agent patient and therapist. Tables 3.1 and 3.2 illustrate a way of addressing these issues. With regard to outcome assessments made by the patient and therapist useful information might be generated by focusing upon the therapist's perception of the patient, and the patient's perception of the therapist. Such an approach to evaluative research in art therapy would at the very least have the merit of not disregarding the patient's perception of therapy in favour of the therapist's, and in so doing provide the latter with a wealth of valuable information about the factors which those with whom they work found most helpful. As Sloane and co-workers note, when discussing their assessments of the therapist–patient relationship in their comparative study of psychotherapy and behaviour therapy, 'In psychotherapy, but not in behaviour therapy, patients who were liked by their therapists showed greater improvement than those who were less liked... Successful patients in both therapies rated the personal inter-action with the therapist as the single most important part of their treatment' (Sloane, Staples, Cristol, Yorkston and Whipple, 1975, p. 225).

If the individual case study ($N = 1$) approach to research were widely adopted by experienced practitioners using system-atic and consistent means for collecting data it would be

Table 3.1: Gathering referral information systematically

Wakefield Health Authority	Name
Stanley Royd Hospital	D.o.B.
	Marital status
	Consultant
	Ward
	Date of admission
	Diagnosis

Art Therapy Referral Form

Please indicate reasons for referral — Tick any of the following you
feel to be appropriate.

☐	Re-build confidence in abilities
☐	Develop awareness of others
☐	Aid memory, attention span and/or concentration
☐	Maintain and improve quality of life
☐	Express feelings
☐	Help gain insight into present difficulties
☐	Increase motivation
☐	Relaxation
☐	Other (Please specify) _____

Please indicate how severe you regard the problem that led to this patient's
admission. Base your opinion on the last month or so and please circle *one*
answer only.

1. Very severely disturbed/ill/upset

2. Moderately severely disturbed/ill/upset

3. In between or don't know

4. Moderately well/recovered/happy

5. Very well/almost completely recovered/very much improved

Please provide any *additional* information you believe should be known about this
patient.

Please state whether a written assessment report will be required, yes/no

If yes, please indicate when required _____

Date _____   Referred by _____

NB. This referral form should *only* be signed by the patient's doctor.

65

Table 3.2: Obtaining the patient's perception of art therapy

Art Therapy — Assessment Form

Name _____ Ward _____

Today's date _____

I would appreciate your help. I want to assess how helpful you found art therapy. Please tick the box you think best describes the helpfulness or unhelpfulness of the following items. Please tick *one* box only for each item.

Item	A lot of help	Some help	In between/ don't know	Not much help	No help
Receiving encouragement and support					
Being able to get off the ward					
Being able to see yourself change					
Discovering your own potential					
The therapist's confidence in your abilities					
Experiencing peace and quiet					
Being able to make a mess					
Being able to try out different materials					
The personality of the therapist					
Being helped to understand your problems					
Being able to express yourself					
The skill of the therapist					

Being able to talk to an understanding person					
Being encouraged to take responsibility for yourself					
Being listened to					
Being able to share your problems with other people					
Being able to relax and enjoy yourself					

Please write any additional comments you may wish to make in the space below.

Thank you for your help.

David Edwards
Senior Art Therapist
Stanley Royd Hospital
Wakefield

possible in a relatively short space of time to obtain a considerable amount of clinically useful information concerning the most potent processes involved in promoting change through art therapy, and provide a much clearer picture regarding who gets selected, who drops out, and who benefits. This would seem particularly important for therapists wishing to develop their therapeutic skills, since some patients appear to improve without the therapist ever being sure of the reasons for this, and in those cases where patients deteriorate there is ample opportunity to attribute 'failure' to such factors as lack of motivation or institutional constraints. Whatever means art therapists employ to evaluate their practice attempting to do so is clearly important, and for a relatively young profession like art therapy an open, flexible and enquiring attitude towards research remains crucial to its vitality and future development. This would seem to be especially important at a time when increasing emphasis is being placed on the accountability of practitioners and the evaluation of health care provision generally.

REFERENCES

Anastasi, A. and Foley, J.P. (1944) 'An Experimental Study of the Drawing Behaviour of Adult Psychotics in Comparison with that of a Normal Control Group', *Journal of Experimental Psychology*, *34*, 169-94

Barlow, D.H., Hayes, S.C. and Nelson, R.O. (1984) *The Scientist Practitioner*, Pergamon, New York

Bergin, A.E. and Lambert, M.J. (1978) 'An Evaluation of Therapeutic Outcomes', in S.L. Garfield and A.E. Bergin, (eds), *Handbook of Psychotherapy and Behavior Change: An Empirical Analysis*, Wiley, New York

Crawford, J.W. (1962) 'Art for the Mentally Retarded: Directed or Creative?', *Bulletin of Art Therapy*, *2*, 67-72

Cunningham-Dax, E. (1953) *Experimental Studies in Psychiatric Art*, Faber & Faber, London

Dalley, T. (1979) 'Art Therapy in Psychiatric Treatment: An Illustrated Case Study', *Art Psychotherapy*, *6*, 257-65

Dalley, T. (1980) 'Assessing the Therapeutic Effects of Art: An Illustrated Case Study', *The Arts in Psychotherapy*, *7*, 11-17

Dalley, T. (ed.) (1984) *Art as Therapy*, Tavistock, London

Edwards, M. (1981) 'Art Therapy Now', *Inscape*, *5*, 18-21

Gantt, L. and Schmal, M. (1974) *Art Therapy: A Bibliography*, George Washington University and National Institute of Mental Health, USA

Henzell, J. (1985) 'The Patient and Doctor Procrustes', Unpublished paper presented at the 11th Triennial Congress of International Society for the Study of Art and Psychopathology, London

Hobson, R.F. and Shapiro, D.A. (1970) 'The Personal Questionnaire as a Method of Assessing Change during Psychotherapy', *British Journal of Psychiatry*, *117*, 623-6

Holtom, R. (1977) 'Measuring Change Attributable to Art Therapy', *Inscape*, No. 15, pp. 34-36

Kwiatkowska, H.Y. (1973) 'Discussion of "Art Therapy: A Diagnostic and Therapeutic Tool"', *International Journal of Psychiatry*, *1*, 21-2

Kwiatkowska, H.Y. (1978) *Family Art Therapy*, Thomas, Illinois

Lehmann, H.E. and Risquez, F.A. (1953) 'The Use of Finger Paintings in the Clinical Evaluation of Psychotic Conditions', *Journal of Mental Science*, *99*, 763-77

Levy, B.I. and Ulman, E. (1974) 'The Effect of Training on Judging Psychopathology from Paintings', *American Journal of Art Therapy*, *14*, 24-5

Liebmann, M. (1981) 'The Many Purposes of Art Therapy', *Inscape*, *5*, 26-8

Malan, D.H. (1973) 'The Outcome Problem in Psychotherapy Research', *Archives of General Psychiatry*, *29*, 719-29

Males, J. (1979) 'Is it Right to Carry Out Scientific Research into Art Therapy?', *Therapy*, 3 May, p. 5

Males, J. (1980) 'Art Therapy: Investigations and Implications',

Inscape, 4, 13-15

Rubin, J.A. (1982) 'Art Therapy: What it is and What it is Not', *American Journal of Art Therapy*, 21, 57-8

Russell-Lacy, S., Robinson, V., Benson, J. and Crange, J. (1979) 'An Experimental Study of Pictures Produced by Acute Schizophrenic Subjects', *British Journal of Psychiatry*, 134, 195-200

Serban, G. (1972) 'A Critical Study of Art Therapy in Treating Psychotic Patients', *Behavioural Neuropsychiatry*, 3, 2-20

Sloane, R.B., Staples, F.R., Cristol, A.H., Yorkston, N.H. and Whipple, K. *'Psychotherapy versus Behavior Therapy'*, Harvard University Press, Cambridge, Mass.

Stott, J. (1985) 'An Examination of Methods Used in Art Therapy with Mentally Handicapped Adults'. Unpublished paper presented at the 11th Triennial Congress of the International Society for the Study of Art and Psychopathology London

Swenson, C.H. (1968) 'Empirical Evaluations of Human Figure Drawings', *Psychological Bulletin*, 70, 20-44

Ulman, E. (1961) 'Art Therapy: Problems of Definition', *Bulletin of Art Therapy*, 1, 10-20

Wadeson, H. (1980) *Art Psychotherapy*, John Wiley & Sons, New York

Waller, D. (1984) 'Submission to the Committee of Inquiry into the Arts and Disabled People by the British Association of Art Therapists', *Inscape*, Summer Issue, pp. 14-16

Watkins, M.M. (1981) 'Six Approaches to the Image in Art Therapy', *Spring*, Annual of Archetypal Psychology and Jungian Thought

Yalom, I.D. (1975) *The Theory and Practice of Group Psychotherapy*, Basic Books, New York

EVALUATION IN PSYCHOLOGY

The following three chapters review and illustrate a range of evaluative research methods as applied in psychology. First Gail Bernstein describes a comprehensive vocational training programme for the developmentally disabled at Goodwill Industries in Denver, Colorado. Clients progress through a gradual approximation to work, ranging from closely controlled simulations at home to community-based jobs with little supervision. A 'quality assurance' evaluation system was instituted to address the key programme questions. Dr Bernstein's chapter focuses upon this evaluation system and particularly upon the programme's success in helping clients to acquire relevant skills and become competitively employed. She concludes that this kind of systematic evaluation not only helps to assess the programme's effectiveness, but that it also represents a form of feedback, affecting staff performance.

In Chapter 5 Peter Higson provides an historial introduction to evaluation in behavioural clinical psychology. His focus then shifts to one of the most widespread applications of behavioural methods, the introduction of a 'token economy' with chronic psychiatric patients. Dr Higson argues that direct observation over extended periods is the most powerful way to evaluate interventions such as the token economy. His case study is based on nine chronic schizophrenic patients and their response to variations in the reinforcement system. The results raise some important ethical issues, which are discussed.

The third and final illustration of evaluation and clinical psychology concerns an adult outpatient clinic. Derek Milne begins by reviewing the 'primary care' literature that is most relevant to this study, but points out that there has been very little research on routine clinical practice, as opposed to specially resourced centres. The outcome evaluation which provides his illustration is based on 25 consecutive referrals, each of whom completed questionnaires before, during and after 3 months of behaviour therapy. The major finding was that those patients who improved seemed to do so because they had developed better coping strategies. Independent ratings made by referring agents corroborated the improvement findings, while patients were satisfied with the service in terms of the dimensions of its process, outcome, content and goals.

4

Evaluation in Clinical/ Occupational Psychology:
Employment Training Programmes for Adults with Developmental Disabilities

Gail Bernstein

4.1 INTRODUCTION

The notion of evaluating human service programmes is of fairly recent origin. It is only in the past 10-20 years that anyone has suggested human service programmes should be evaluated in order to determine whether they are accomplishing what they are supposed to be accomplishing (Gurel, 1975). This lack of attention to evaluation comes as no surprise, for the prevalent attitude on the part of both human service professionals and other members of society has been that human services are doing good things and the judgement of professionals should be relied on to tell citizens whether in fact the services they pay for are doing good things. The lack of interest in evaluation of developmental disabilities services is no doubt due partly to this general social lack of interest in evaluation. However, it is also due in part to the historical lack of expectations that persons with developmental disabilities would change significantly as a result of service provision. Rather, the prevailing assumption was that services were primarily devoted to a caretaking and maintenance function.

In the past 15 years the emphasis in services for persons with developmental disabilities has shifted radically from the care-taking and maintenance assumption to the habilitation and education assumption. That is, we now assume services will result in clear, significant changes in the life of an individual receiving them. This change in emphasis is perhaps most pronounced with respect to vocational services. Specifically, it is now clear that, given proper services, most of the people served in programmes for the developmentally disabled can in fact be gainfully employed, many in jobs paying competitive wages or better. The present chapter is devoted to an examination of evaluation of employment training programmes for persons with developmental disabilities as it has been reported in the published literature, to one detailed example of such an evaluation, and to recommendations for the future.

4.2 CURRENT PRACTICE IN EVALUATION OF EMPLOYMENT TRAINING PROGRAMMES

Until fairly recently the primary sources of evaluation data on employment training and placement for persons with disabilities in the United States have been reports from state rehabilitation agencies.

Major limitations of these data are that no specific placement model has usually been practised, and that a successful placement is typically defined as one where a person is still employed after 60-90 days on the job. In fact 'there is no literature that we are familiar with which focuses directly on one placement model and its record of success over time with a given pool of disabled persons' (Hill, Hill, Wehman et al., 1985, p. 68).

Given these deficiencies in existing literature, recent authors in employment training for persons with developmental disabilities have taken a somewhat different approach. Published reports on employment training programmes have increased dramatically in number in the past 10 years, and no attempt will be made here to review comprehensively that literature. Instead, three programmes have been chosen which are well known and which have published extensive descriptions of their programmes, and data on the results. The choice of these three programmes is in no way meant as a criticism of the many other excellent programmes currently in existence.

The programmes which form the basis for the discussion that follows are: the food service training programme at the University of Washington (Moss, 1979; Ford, Dineen and Hall, in press); the Mid-Nebraska Training Programs (Schalock and Lilley, in press; Schalock and Harper, 1978; Schalock, 1983) and the work of Wehman and his colleagues in Virginia (Wehman and Hill, 1985; Wehman, 1981, and Wehman and

Hill, 1982). These three programmes have several characteristics in common. First, they all use behavioural training strategies to teach employment skills; strategies that have been validated through single-subject research. Second, they all use on-the-job training, some subsequent to other training and some as the primary form of training. Finally, all of them provide and assume the necessity of providing indefinite follow-along support for employed graduates of their programmes. These common features have been found to be basic to all of the currently successful employment training programmes described in recent literature (Rudrud, Ziarnik, Bernstein and Ferrera, 1984).

There is remarkable agreement among these three programmes on the use of basic descriptive and evaluative measures. All report descriptive information on those served, which includes: age, sex, intelligence level, types and numbers of disabilities, employment training history, living situation and referral source. Further, all report outcome measures, which include: whether or not the individual is competitively employed, hourly wages, gross wages (and, by implication, hours worked), type of job, job retention (i.e. length of employment), and variables related to job retention.

Other measures reported by one or two of these programmes include: quality of life, family support characteristics, specific skills gained during training, and a variety of measures of the cost of training. The implication here is that there is considerable agreement as to the desired outcomes of these programmes; namely, that they result in increases in the types of jobs held, the wages earned and job retention as a result of programme service. There has been less emphasis to date on process measures such as skills gained during training.

4.3. PROGRAMME EVALUATION AT GOODWILL–DENVER

Since February 1982 the author and her colleagues have been involved with the rehabilitation programme at Goodwill Industries in Denver, Colorado (Ziarnik, 1983; Rudrud et al., 1984).

This programme focuses primarily on teaching generic work skills needed to obtain and maintain employment in a variety of settings (e.g. response to instruction, staying on task). At entry,

73

the trainee's present level of behaviour is assessed using the Worker Skills Checklist (WSC) (Ziarnik, Grupe, Morrison *et al.*, 1983). The Checklist is based on the literature on factors related to vocational success, and was subsequently socially validated by surveying local employers.

The first programme level occurs in house, with individualised programmes intended to promote the acquisition and limited generalisation of the 27 generic work skills listed on the WSC while the trainee engages in simulated work. Single-subject data are collected and graphed for all individualised programmes. Once trainees can engage in the generic work behaviours without the support of artificial consequences such as tokens they move to less supervised, community-based job sites located in actual business. The focus on programmes in the community sites is on self-management of work skills and maintenance of skills with naturally occurring levels of antecedents and consequences. Once trainees can maintain generic work behaviours under normal employment conditions, we provide job placement, on-the-job training, and follow-along support.

When we designed that programme, one of our first tasks was to design an evaluation system which answered the questions that were important for the type of programme we wanted. The design of that evaluation system was conceptualised as part of an integrated quality assurance system. There are four major steps in designing an integrated quality assurance system, as shown in Figure 4.1. The first one is that we must clearly define the goals of the programme. In the case of the Goodwill programme, our goal is to teach people the skills they need in order to obtain and maintain competitive employment and to provide whatever additional supports are needed besides skill development to achieve that goal.

The second step in system design is to use the statement of

Figure 4.1: Designing an integrated quality assurance system

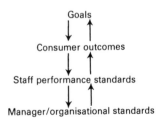

Goals

Consumer outcomes

Staff performance standards

Manager/organisational standards

programme goals specifically to define measurable consumer outcomes that will result from or lead to goal achievement. The measurement of these outcomes then becomes the basis for designing a programme evaluation system. At Goodwill, outcomes fell into two categories. First there are the outcomes that are the results of achieving the goals. These include whether or not individuals obtain competitive employment; how much they are making both on an hourly basis and on a bi-weekly basis; and who is achieving those outcomes in terms of age, sex, disability, ethnic status and other descriptors. A second set of outcomes has to do with the skills needed to obtain and maintain competitive employment. Specifically, 27 exit criteria were identified which a review of the research literature and a survey of local employers indicated are a requirement for successful employment (Ziarnik *et al.*, 1983). Thus the acquisition of those skills was seen as part of the desirable outcomes of the Goodwill programme.

The next step in defining a quality assurance system is the development of staff performance standards. The essential question which must be answered in order to develop performance standards is the following: what must staff do in order to help consumers to achieve the desired outcomes? This step in designing a quality assurance system is a particularly difficult one to accomplish effectively. Too often, staff performance standards are set based on a particular training experience or professional bias of the supervisor or manager, rather than on any empirical reference to what really works in achieving consumer outcomes and what does not. While there is by no means enough information available to base every single staff performance standard on demonstrated effectiveness in achieving consumer outcomes, there is enough evidence to define at least some standards in those terms.

The final step in designing a quality assurance system is to develop managerial and organisational standards which are designed to develop and maintain staff performance which results in desired consumer outcomes. Too often, organisational standards are developed for a variety of reasons that have nothing to do with what is effective in supporting staff behaviour and what is not. Again, while the data are by no means complete, there is enough information available to identify critically needed components of manager and organisational standards.

The focus of the current chapter is on the evaluation system, so that staff performance standards and managerial and organisational standards will not be addressed further. Rather, they are mentioned in order to provide the context for the evaluation system. Additional information will be available in a forthcoming paper (Bernstein and Ziarnik, in preparation). The programme evaluation system for the Goodwill programme is described in Figure 4.2. The system is designed to collect important data about the programme and to meet Commission on the Accreditation of Rehabilitation Facilities (CARF) requirements for programme evaluation. In addition to the regularly collected data, the end-of-year report also reviews and discusses programme goals through the year. The forms staff use to report quarterly data are shown in Figures 4.3-4.5, and the codes used to fill them out are shown in Figure 4.6.

These codes and forms were designed with the help of a computer consultant. Currently the system is programmed on the mainframe computer at the University of Colorado Health

Figure 4.2: Rehabilitation programme evaluation at Goodwill

Purpose	The aim of an effective programme evaluation system is two-fold: to tell the programme staff what they are doing well and what needs improvement; and tell programme staff, administrators, boards of directors, and interested members of the community what the programme is doing for the people it serves.
Programme goal	The training programme at Goodwill Industries of Denver is designed to teach developmentally disabled individuals the skills needed to gain and maintain competitive employment.
Responsibility	The programme evaluation system and reports on it are the responsibility of the Rehabilitation Director. That individual delegates evaluation duties as needed.
Frequency	An evaluation report is prepared within 4 weeks after the end of each quarter. A yearly compilation is also prepared at the end of each calendar year.
Dissemination	Evaluation reports are sent to the President, Board of Directors, and Rehabilitation Staff. Reports will also be available to interested members of the community.

Report contents	Population served
	    Demographics (age, sex, disability, time at Goodwill,
	        number served, ethnicity)
	Outcomes
	    Status changes (e.g. to TEPS sites, to competitive
	        employment)
	    Follow-up (maintenance in employment)
	Process
	    Proactivity
	    Quality of individual objective programmes
	    Progress on objectives

		Attendance
		Earnings
		Staff satisfaction/burnout
	Dissemination	
		Tours
		Internships
Evaluation process	1.	*Rehabilitation staff* are informed that it is time for a quarterly evaluation and asked to complete trainee progress reports for (1) all trainees on their caseloads as of the day the reports are completed, and (2) all trainees who withdrew during the quarter being evaluated and were on their caseloads at the time of withdrawal. Rehabilitation staff also complete trainee entry reports for all trainees who entered during the quarter being evaluated.
	2.	The *Rehabilitation Director* administers the Staff Satisfaction Scale and the Staff Burnout Scale to all rehabilitation staff.
	3.	The *Evaluator* rates four objective plans written by each case manager during the quarter, using the rating checklist.
	4.	The *Evaluator* examines files of all trainees for whom no objectives exist.
	5.	The *Evaluator* collects follow-up information on employed former trainees from all staff with follow-up responsibilities.
	6.	The *Evaluator* scores both satisfaction measures.
	7.	The *Evaluator* transfers all trainee data from the completed forms to the computer and prepares the quarterly report.

Sciences Center. Within the year we hope to acquire a micro-computer and transfer the system to it. The goal is to have all forms programmed as screens which staff can call up and use to enter data directly. The program for this system does require a relational data base. We are currently reviewing available soft-ware to determine which packages will meet our needs.

The Checklist for Evaluating Behavior Change Programs is shown in Figure 4.7. It was originally developed for use during a statewide study of staff training needs (Bernstein, 1981). We have found it to be extremely valuable both for establishing expectations for staff performance in writing behaviour change programmes and for assessing that performance. We evaluated inter-observer agreement for the data presented here by rating nine programmes out of the total number rated between 1982 through 1984. Each was rated separately by the author and the then programme director, Dr Jon Ziarnik. Agreement range was 73-100 and mean agreement was 90 per cent.

Figure 4.3: Trainee entry report

Soc. Sec. # ☐☐☐ ☐☐ ☐☐☐☐ First Initial Middle Initial

Name ☐☐☐☐☐☐☐☐☐☐☐☐☐☐☐☐ ☐ ☐

Date of Birth ☐☐ ☐☐ ☐☐ Ethnicity ☐ (C, B, H, N, A, U)

GW Entry Date ☐☐ ☐☐ ☐☐ Sex ☐ M ☐ F

Case Manager ☐☐

Referral Source ☐☐☐ (CCB, DPS, PRI, SLF, OTH, CDR)

Disabilities (four maximum) ☐☐☐☐ MIMR EPIL OTHR
☐☐☐☐ MDMR CERP
☐☐☐☐ SEMR PSYC
☐☐☐☐ PRMR SPIM
HRIM
VIIM
ORIM
ALCO
LDIS

Status at Entry ☐☐☐ INH, TEP, OTH

Staff satisfaction is measured as part of the regular programme evaluation system, but will not be addressed further here, as the purpose of this chapter is to address client issues. However, we strongly recommend ongoing attention to staff satisfaction as part of any quality assurance effort.

4.4   OUTCOMES AT GOODWILL–DENVER

Tables 4.1 and 4.2 give descriptive information about persons served in the Goodwill–Denver programme for 1982-5 (all data are complete through 1 October 1985). The two noticeable changes in those served have been in length of time in programme and disabilities of those served. In the first quarter of 1982 the people served averaged 1.35 disabilities per person. In the third quarter of 1985 the average was 1.47 disabilities per person. Thus the population currently served displays more multiple disabilities than in past years. Also, the number served with speech or visual impairments has increased, as has the number with severe mental retardation.

Figure 4.4: Trainee quarterly report

Soc. Sec. #

Client Name

Reporting Period — Quarter (1, 2, 3, 4)

First Initial — Middle Initial

Current Programme Manager

Status Changes During Quarter (If Any)

New Status — Date of Change

Programme Manager Change During Quarter (If Any)

New Programme Manager — Date of Change

Days Absent for Quarter — Days Inactive for Quarter

Follow-up or OJT Hours for Quarter

Type of Job, if Employed

Objective Status (report on all objectives except those completed or discontinued prior to first day of quarter being reported)

Objective Code	Start Date	Direction (I, D, M)	Status (P, C, D, N, M)	Date Completed or Discontinued

Figure 4.5: Wages report

Month ———————— Year ————————

Last Name	Initial	S.S. #	Pay Date	Gross Pay	Hourly	Pay Date	Gross Pay	Hourly

Figure 4.6: Codes and definitions for data system

I. Referral Source

CCB — Community Center Board
DPS — Denver Public Schools
CDR — Colorado Division of Rehabilitation
PRI — Private
SLF — Self
OTH — Other

II. Disabilities

MIMR — Mild Mental Retardation
MDMR — Moderate Mental Retardation
SEMR — Severe Mental Retardation
PRMR — Profound Mental Retardation
LDIS — Learning Disability
EPIL — Epilepsy
CERP — Cerebral Palsy
PSYC — Psychiatric Impairment
SPIM — Speech Impairment
HRIM — Hearing Impairment
VIIM — Visual Impairment
ORIM — Orthopaedic Impairment
ALCO — Alcoholism
OTHR — Other

III. Status

INH — In House
TEP — Transitional Employment Site
WDR — Withdrew from Goodwill
TRM — Terminated by Goodwill
EMP — Competitively Employed
FEM — Fired from Competitive Employment
REM — Resigned from Competitive Employment
OTH — Other (Includes Rehab OJT)
SJT — Specialised Job Training
LOF — Laid Off
OPO — Other Positive Outcome
JTP — JTPA Grant Trainee
CAR — Caregiver Grant Trainee
DEC — Deceased
EMB, EMC — Second, third job for Graduate
of Programme
ESA, ESB, ESC, etc. — First, second, etc., job
for former Trainee who
left before graduation

IV. Case Manager

00 — Anyone not listed below
01 — K. Conway   09 — K. Pantzer
02 — J. Leeming   10 — M. Miller
03 — R. Grupe   11 — J. Gorman
04 — N. Cruchon   12 — D. Smith
05 — J. Drain   13 — R. Wagner
06 — R. Kellerman   14 — G. Rogers
07 — V. Potestivo   15 — J. Johnson

Figure 4.6 continued

08 — B. Albracht   16 — K. Freundlich
                       17 — D. Calderwood
                       18 — N. Laughlin

V.   Ethnicity

C — Caucasian   N — Native American
B — Black   A — Asian
H — Hispanic   U — Unknown

VI.   Objectives

For each objective, identify it with the code for
the relevant exit criterion from the list
attached, followed by the number indicating how
many objectives this client has had for that exit
criterion. For instance, the second objective
an individual has had related to calling in
absences would be A CALL 2.

See attached list of exit criteria and codes
for them.

VII.   Status

P — Progress Being Made   C — Completed
D — Discontinued   N — No Programme
M — Maintaining

Note: For objectives achieved which then become maintenance objectives,
proceed as in the following example:

If WONTK 01 was completed, code it C and give the date of
completion. Call the maintenance objective WONTK 02 and code it M
as long as the behaviour maintains and the objective continues.

VIII.   Inactive days — all planned days out and, in the case of a legitimate
           medical absence of 3 or more consecutive days, all
           days except the first 2.

IX.   Follow-up or OJT hours — Staff time spent following
           trainees who are no
           longer in in-house or TEP
           status. This includes
           travel time.

Attendance

ATEND   1. Attends 21 out of 22 possible working days per month.
ACALL   2. Calls in all absences to supervisor within 10 minutes of the
            beginning of the work day.
AAPTS   3. Plans and communicates any work day appointments with
            supervisor in accordance with company policy.
AVACA   4. Plans and communicates vacation time within acceptable company
            policy.
ATRNS   5. Reaches work place by means of own arrangement (bus, taxi,
            bike).
APNCH   6. Punches in and out 100% of time.
APRMT   7. Is at work station on time.

Work Skills

WMATS   8. Only brings appropriate work or break materials to work. All non-work materials stored in designated area.

WSTRT   9. Gets out work materials and begins work immediately.

WDURA 10. Works at assigned task continuously for 1 hour and 50 minutes.

WONTK 11. Is on task 95% of the time observed (*must* look busy).

WPROD 12. Maintains a consistent 85% productivity rate (waived with physical handicap).

WCLEN 13. Cleans up work area at the end of the day.

WRULS 14. Follows company rules as instructed.

WGROM 15. Keeps body clean and odour free.

WIDEN 16. Communicates upon request:

     a. Full name
     b. Address
     c. Home telephone

WNEDS 17. Manages production needs appropriately by either communicating with supervisor or independently getting more materials within 5 seconds of running out of materials.

Social Skills

SNEDS 18. Communicates basic needs that may interfere with ability to continue working such as sickness, pain, or when cannot do job and needs help.

SINST   19. When given an instruction:

     a. Makes eye contact
     b. Gives verbal acknowledgment with normal voice tone
     c. Has neutral or pleasant facial expression.
     d. Complies within 5 seconds

SCOMP 20. Responds to an instruction that requires compliance after a specified time interval.

SCORR   21. When work performance is corrected by any person identified as authority:

     a. Makes eye contact
     b. Gives verbal acknowledgment with normal voice tone
     c. Has neutral or pleasant facial expression
     d. Corrects mistake within 5 seconds

SPRAS 22. When praised gives verbal acknowledgment in pleasant tone and returns to work.

SEXPR 23. Express interpersonal issues or feelings appropriate to work place in a socially approved manner.

SCOOP 24. Gets along (e.g., cooperation, pleasant, etc.) with co-workers without prompts.

SINTR   25. Seeks out and initiates interaction appropriate to work place with other workers during breaks at least 4 times/week.

STRTH 26. Relates verifiable facts.

SPOSS 27. Has only personal or approved items in possession.

Long-Term Maintenance Objectives

MWAIT — Waiting for placement at next level
MINAP — Inappropriately placed, being referred out
MOTHR — Other

From: Rudrud, EH., Ziarnik, J.P., Bernstein, G.S. & Ferrara J.M. (1984). *Proactive Vocational Habilitation.* Paul H. Brookes Publishing Co.; Baltimore. Reprinted by permission.)

Figure 4.7: Checklist for evaluating behavior change programs

	Rating	(For all items 0 = not stated at all)
Behavior Is the target behavior stated?		3 = observable and measurable 2 = observable (behavioral) not measurable 1 = neither
Is the current behavior stated?		3 = observable and measurable 2 = observable, not measurable 1 = neither
Rationale Is the target behavior necessary to meet one of the WRC criteria?		3 = WRC criterion explicitly identified 2 = target is connected to WRC, but connection not explicitly stated 1 = neither — some other rationale
Conditions Does the program specify where it will be implemented?		3 = specific room or program 1 = not specific room or program
Does the program specify when it will be implemented (time and days or week)?		3 = times and days 2 = one of the above 1 = neither
Does the program specify who is responsible for implementation?		3 = name or position title if only one with that title 1 = not name or position title if only one with that title
Method Does the program specify what to do before the behavior occurs?		3 = can do from reading 2 = behavioral not enough to do 1 = not behavioral
Does the program specify consequences? Contingencies (schedule)?		3 = can do from reading 2 = behavioral, not enough to do 1 = not behavioral
Measurement Does the program indicate when data are to be collected?		3 = times and days 2 = one of the above 1 = neither
Is the recording procedure described?		3 = can do from reading 2 = behavioral but not enough to do 1 = not behavioral
Is the behavior being measured stated?		3 = observable and measurable 2 = observable but not measurable or osb/msb. but includes target criteria 1 = neither observable nor measurable

Data Summaries Is the unit of time identified?	3 = actual dates or similar ID for other units 1 = any other time identification
Are the behaviors being measured identified?	3 = observable descriptive label 1 = any other identification
Are the treatment conditions clearly identified?	3 = labelled and separated 2 = labelled or separated, not both 1 = any other reference to treatment conditions
The most recent data entry is no more than two weeks old	3 = yes 2 = more than 2 weeks, less than 4 1 = more than 4 weeks
Evaluation Does the program specify who is responsible for review of the data?	3 = person or position if only one with that title 1 = not person or position if only one with that title
Does the program specify when the reviews are to occur?	3 = 2 weeks or less 2 = more than 2 weeks but no more than 1 month 1 = more than 1 month apart
Are the behavioral criteria and/or the conditions under which behavior occurs changed when the previous standard is met? (skill acquisition programs only)	3 = changed after no more than 10, no less than 5 successive data points at standard 2 = changed after more than 10, less than 16 1 = all other

Source: Gail S. Bernstein, Jon P. Ziarnik, Eric H. Rudrud; Goodwill Version — 2/85 Revision

Current programme status as of 1 October 1985 of everyone served in 1982-5 is shown in Table 4.3. There were 26 programme graduates employed. These 26 individuals represent a 74 per cent maintenance rate: that is, we have graduated 35 persons into employment since 1982, of whom 26 are still employed. Of these, 14 were referred to us by the developmental disabilities system, 11 by the state rehabilitation agency, and 1 by the public schools. Table 4.4 describes these individuals in terms of age, ethnic background, sex, and disabilities. Types of jobs held, number of jobs, months employed, and months in the programme are shown in Table 4.5. The only person listed who earns less than minimum wage is the contracts employee at Goodwill, who is paid on a piece-rate basis. Average hourly and

Table 4.1: Age, sex, time in programme, and ethnicity of persons served, 1982–5

	1982 Quarter			1983 Quarter				1984 Quarter				1985 Quarter		
	2	3	4	1	2	3	4	1	2	3	4	1	2	3
Number served	72	64	67	67	70	75	77	83	89	84	89	88	94	90
Mean age	33	33	33	31	33	32	33	a	31	32	32	32	32	32
Sex														
Men	41	37	39	41	41	41	42	49	53	46	48	52	53	52
Women	30	27	28	26	29	34	35	34	36	38	41	36	41	38
Mean months in Goodwill programme	a	31	30	30	30	29	30	a	29	34	34	35	35	40
Ethnicity														
Asian									2	2	2	2	2	2
Black									14	11	12	11	13	13
Caucasian									64	63	65	66	68	62
Hispanic									9	8	10	9	10	10
Native American									0	0	0	0	0	1
Unknown									0	0	0	0	1	2

Note: ethnicity was not tallied prior to second quarter, 1984.
a Not tallied for this quarter

Table 4.2: Disabilities of persons served, 1982–5

	1982 Quarter			1983 Quarter				1984 Quarter				1985 Quarter		
	2	3	4	1	2	3	4	1	2	3	4	1	2	3
Mental retardation														
Mild	37	29	33	38	39	43	42	49	53	59	53	51	57	55
Moderate	16	21	20	22	21	21	19	13	16	14	15	15	17	16
Severe	3	2	6	4	4	3	4	5	5	6	6	7	7	8
Profound	0	0	0	0	0	0	0	1	1	1	1	1	1	0
Epilepsy	10	8	9	10	11	13	12	18	16	16	17	12	13	13
Cerebral palsy	3	5	5	3	2	3	3	2	1	1	1	2	2	5
Psychiatric impairment	7	4	6	3	4	4	3	4	3	5	5	8	8	7
Speech impairment	2	0	0	1	2	2	1	6	6	7	5	7	7	5
Hearing impairment	3	2	3	1	4	4	3	4	4	4	3	3	4	4
Visual impairment	3	3	3	0	3	2	6	8	8	9	7	7	9	9
Orthopaedic impairment	6	2	2	1	3	2	2	2	1	0	0	0	0	0
Alcoholism	1	1	1	0	0	2	2	2	2	2	2	2	2	2
Other	6	2	5	2	3	5	4	10	9	10	7	10	8	8
Total disabilities	97[a]	79[b]	93	85	96	106	101	124	125	124	123	125	135	132
Total served	72	64	67	67	70	75	77	83	89	84	89	88	94	90

[a]Does not include three with unknown level of mental retardation.
[b]Does not include two with unknown level of mental retardation.

Table 4.3: Program status as of 1 October 1985 for persons served, 1982-5

Programme graduates	
Employed	26
Resigned from employment	2
Fired from employment	2
Deceased	1
Specialised job training	3
Other positive outcome	1
Current trainees	
Transitional employment	26
In-house training	34
Other former trainees	
Fired from employment	3
Withdrew	43
Terminated by programme	38

Table 4.4: Age, ethnicity, sex and disabilities, of Goodwill graduates employed as of 1 October 1985

Age	Ethnicity	Sex	Disabilities
25	C	M	MDMR
30	C	M	MDMR, SPIM
39	C	F	MIMR, ALCO
29	B	F	MIMR
28	H	F	MIMR
41	C	M	MIMR
59	C	F	EPIL
41	C	M	MIMR, EPIL
54	C	M	MIMR
27	C	F	MIMR, HRIM
26	B	F	MIMR
54	C	M	MIMR, SPIM, HRIM
35	C	M	MIMR
49	B	M	MDMR
44	C	F	MIMR, ALCO
22	C	M	MIMR, EPIL
27	B	F	MIMR
41	B	F	MIMR, HRIM, VIIM
25	H	M	MIMR
44	C	F	MIMR, EPIL, VIIM
26	A	M	EPIL
31	C	M	MIMR
29	C	M	MIMR
24	C	M	MIMR
33	H	F	MIMR, PSYC
32	C	F	borderline MR

Acronyms are explained in section II of Figure 4.6.

Table 4.5: Current job, number of jobs, months employed, months in programme for Goodwill graduates currently employed

Current job	Number of jobs since graduation	Months employed since graduation	Months in programmes prior to graduation
Houskeeping	2	27	6
Runner–Goodwill	2	6	128[a]
Janitor	2	34	7
Dishwasher	2	19	2
Food preparer	2	12	17
Pallet marker	3	36	18[a]
Clotheshanger–Goodwill	1	17	2
Stocker	1	8	11
Dishwasher	1	5	42[a]
Shirt presser	1	11	24
Headset wrapper	1	33	8
Contracts worker–Goodwill	1	3	49[a]
Collections attendant–Goodwill	1	15	3
Headset washer	1	32	40[a]
Pricer–Goodwill	1	15	36
Headset processing worker	1	11	13
Busperson	1	2	29
Janitor	1	4	14
Electronics assembler	1	6	29
Janitor–Goodwill	1	9	19
Runner–Goodwill	1	2	32
Stablehand	1	9	9
Janitor	1	11	15
Dishwasher	1	12	8
Busperson	1	6	9
Clotheshanger–Goodwill	1	18	1

[a]This includes time in programme prior to 1982, doing sheltered contract work.

bi-weekly wages for the third quarter of 1985 are shown in Table 4.6 for all transitional and competitive employees. In addition, 24 of the 26 get paid vacation — eight get 1 week a year, the rest get 2 weeks a year. Twenty of the 26 have health insurance available — six major medical and 14 comprehensive coverage.

Process measures are shown in Table 4.7. Three questions are asked about programme process: what proportion of individualised objectives are proactive (i.e. designed to increase or maintain behaviour), how well are trainees progressing on their

Table 4.6: Earnings for third quarter, 1985 ($US)

Status	Average gross hourly wage	Average gross biweekly wages
Employed, third job	4.68	246.11
Employed, second job	4.21	329.49
Employed, first job	3.15	212.39
Transitional employment	1.05	63.86

objectives, and how well-written are the objectives? On this last measure, quality of objectives, all staff are expected to maintain ratings of at least 90 per cent on all objectives they write.

4.4 CONTRIBUTIONS OF THE GOODWILL EVALUATION SYSTEM

This extensive data set makes several major contributions to the existing literature. First, it adds to the rapidly growing evidence that persons with developmental disabilities can, given effective training, become competitively employed. This is hardly news to anyone who is familiar with the programmes cited earlier. However, the technology and philosophy that result in competitive employment are still exceptions to the norm in the majority of service delivery programmes. Hence the more successes of programmes such as the one at Goodwill, the more compelling the case for such programmes becomes.

Second, the extensive descriptive data allow accurate comparisons between (1) outcomes of the Goodwill programme and outcomes of other employment training programmes, and (2) current, past, and future outcomes of the Goodwill programme.

The third major contribution this report makes to our knowledge base is that it explicitly defines and measures programme quality. The Checklist for Evaluating Behavior Change Programs is the centrepiece of the programme quality measures. It is important because it focuses on process, not technique; hence it will not become outmoded as our technical sophistication increases. Further, and most important, it sets standards which foster behaviour analysts rather than behaviour technicians (e.g. if something hasn't worked for 10 consecutive data points, drop it and try something else).

Implicit in this focus on programme quality as a process

Table 4.7: Process Measures for Goodwill programme, 1982–5

	1982 Quarter			1983 Quarter				1984 Quarter				1985 Quarter		
	2	3	4	1	2	3	4	1	2	3	4	1	2	3
Total objectives	139	117	86	116	125	128	117	115	111	121	102	105	136	143
Percentage to increase behaviour	86	95	97	86	85	80	82	96	97	87	83	87	86	73
Percentage to maintain behaviour	9	4	2	9	14	16	15	3	3	9	16	13	12	27
Progress														
Percentage met	27	34	33	33	40	26	22	17	10	11	16	19	12	22
Percentage progress made	56	48	50	60	49	59	62	65	62	52	61	61	53	45
Percentage maintained									6	8	11	10	12	20
Percentage discontinued									18	25	13	10	14	14
Quality														
Mean percentage of total possible	48	75	84	93	95	94	94	94	93	93	91	97	97	91

Note: Separate maintained and discontinued percentages for progress were not kept prior to the second quarter of 1984.

measure is the notion that evaluation is not simply a means of assessing programme outcome, but is also an intervention in its own right. More specifically, given the strong and consistent effects of regular feedback on staff performance (e.g. Bernstein, 1982, 1984), it is clear that any evaluation conducted within an organisation in which the results are regularly reported to people implementing the programme, is certain to serve as an intervention as well as an evaluation. Given that this is likely to occur, it is remarkable how little attention has been paid in published evaluation reports to describing how often, and in what form, staff receive the data from programme evaluations and what, if any, are the effects of those reports on staff performance. (For a more detailed discussion of this issue, see Bernstein and Ziarnik, in preparation.)

Finally, the presentation of the evaluation forms and procedures provides an example of a comprehensive programme evaluation system which can be used to obtain summary data in employment training programmes. This is important because most programmes serving persons with developmental disabilities are used to documenting progress in terms of individuals, not aggregate data, and/or are often not used to being accountable for outcomes such as employment. Further, since practitioners often object to the time required for data collection, examples of efficient ways to collect information are badly needed. The major time investment in the system presented here was in its design (forms, computer program, schedule). Ongoing implementation requires only a small time investment from each staff member on an infrequent basis.

4.5   FUTURE DIRECTIONS

Evaluation in employment training programmes for adults with developmental disabilities has been notable more for impressiveness of outcomes than for sophistication of methodology. In fact, it is likely that the effectiveness of published programmes has been so clear (i.e. people who have never been competitively employed getting and keeping jobs), there has been little impetus for increased rigour.

There are two ways in which current evaluation methods are lacking and do need development. One has to do with measurement. The most basic measure to date has been competitive employment. However, current initiatives are emphasising supported employment, defined as (1) paid employment, which (2) provides daily social interactions with people without disabilities who are not paid service providers, and (3) which provides publicly funded ongoing support directly related to sustaining employment (Bellamy and Melia, 1984). This implies that the desirable vocational outcome for some individuals receiving services is not full competitive employment without ongoing support. If so, additional measures are needed which allow us to measure supported employment outcomes. Specifically, we need measures of integration and of support (e.g. type, amount) as well as the measures already in place of gross and hourly wages and hours worked. Use of measures of integration and support is critical to distinguishing between supported employment and sheltered workshops.

The second area where increased methodological sophistication is needed is analysis of programme methodology in relation to individual needs and outcomes. Schalock and his colleagues have begun work in one aspect of this area, goodness-of-fit between persons and their environments (Schalock and Jensen, in press). In general, we need to know how to achieve the best results for the widest variety of individuals in the most efficient manner. Examples of questions which might be addressed are: What types of support result in the greatest job retention, and are different types of support needed for different individuals? Who is most likely to benefit from receiving all training on-the-job, and who is most likely to benefit from training prior to placement in the job setting? What staff resources are needed, in which environments, to produce optimal results?

The challenge to professionals working in employment training programmes is to retain the existing emphasis on important outcomes while meeting current needs for additional measures and analysis of effective methodologies. A continued commitment to an experimental orientation is the foundation for meeting this challenge.

ACKNOWLEDGEMENTS

From 1982 through 1984 the Goodwill programme described in this chapter was directed by my good friend and former colleague, Dr Jon P. Ziarnik. No report on the programme would be complete without an acknowledgement of his efforts, the contributions of our skilled and energetic staff, and the support of the Goodwill administration, particularly Tim Welker, President of Goodwill Industries of Denver.

REFERENCES

Bellamy, G.T. and Melia, R. (1984) Memorandum to Participants in OSERS Planning Meeting on Supported Employment. US Department of Education, Washington, DC, 9 May

Bernstein, G.S. (1981) *Staff Development for Providers of Service to Developmentally Delayed Disabled Persons: Planning for the Future.* John F. Kennedy Child Development Center, Denver

Bernstein, G.S. (1982). 'Training Behavior Change Agents: A Conceptual Review', *Behavior Therapy, 13,* 1-23

Bernstein, G.S. (1984). Training of Behavior Change Agents, in M. Hersen, R.N. Eisler, and P.M. Miller (eds), *Progress in Behavior Modification,* vol. 17, Academic Press, New York

Bernstein, G.S. and Ziarnik, J.P. (In preparation) 'Quality Assurance in a Vocational Habilitation Program'

Ford, L., Dineen, J. and Hall, J. (In press) 'Is there Life after Placement?', *Education and Training of the Mentally Retarded*

Gurel, L. (1975) 'The Human Side of Evaluating Human Services Programs: Problems and Prospects', in: M. Gutentaug and E.L. Struening (eds), *Handbook of Evaluation Research,* vol. II, Sage, Beverly Hills, Calif.

Hill, J.W., Hill, M., Wehman, P., Banks, P.D., Pendleton, P. and Britt, C. (1985) 'Demographic Analysis Related to Successful Job Retention for Competitively Employed Persons who are Mentally Retarded', in *Competititve Employment for Persons with Mental Retardation: From Research to Practice,* vol. I, Rehabilitation Research and Training Center, Richmond, Virginia

Moss, J.W. (1979). *Post-secondary Vocational Education for Mentally Retarded Adults.* ERIC Clearing House on Handicapped Gifted Children, Reston, VA

O'Neill, C. (1984) 'Employment Data: What Information to Keep and How to Use it. Presented at 'Better Wages: Better Jobs for Persons with Developmental Disabilities', a vocational conference, Copper Mountain, Col.

Rudrud, E.H., Ziarnik, J.P., Bernstein, G.S. and Ferrera, J.M. (1984) *Proactive Vocational Habilitation,* Paul Brookes, Baltimore, Md.

Schalock, R.L. (1983) *Services for Developmental Disabled Adults: Development, Implementation and Evaluation,* University Park Press, Baltimore, Md.

Schalock, R.L. and Harper, R.S. (1978) 'Placement from Community-based Mental Retardation Programs: How Well do Clients Do?',

American Journal of Mental Deficiency, 83, 240-7

Schalock, R.L. and Jensen, C.M. (In press) 'Assessing the Goodness of Fit between Persons and their Environments', *Journal of the Association for Persons with Severe Handicaps*

Schalock, R.L. and Lilley, M.A. (In press) 'Placement from Community-based Mental Retardation Programs: How Well do Clients do after 8 to 10 years?', *American Journal of Mental Deficiency*

Wehman, P. (1981) *Competitive Employment: New Horizons for Severely Disabled Individuals,* Paul Brookes, Baltimore, Md.

Wehman, P. and Hill, J.W. (1985) *Competitive Employment for Persons with Mental Retardation: From Research to Practice,* vol. I, Rehabilitation Research and Training Center, Richmond, Va.

Wehman, P. and Hill, M. (1982) *Vocational Training and Placement of Severely Disabled Persons,* vol. III, Commonwealth University, Richmond, Va.

Ziarnik, J.P. (Chairman) (1983) *Disseminating Behavioral Technology: Program Engineering in a Vocational Training Agency.* Group poster session presented at the meeting of the Association for Behavior Analysis, Milwaukee

Ziarnik, J.P., Grupe, R., Morrison, C., Cruchon, C., Conway, K. and Leeming, J. (1983) 'Worker Skills Checklist', unpublished manuscript, Goodwill Industries of Denver

5

Evaluation in Clinical Psychology:
Evaluating Behavioural Interventions in Psychiatric Hospitals

Peter Higson

5.1 INTRODUCTION

The history of the application of behavioural principles goes hand in hand with the development and refinement of single-case research designs (e.g. Hersen and Barlow, 1976; Kazdin, 1982a). For several reasons this methodology is more suitable for evaluating the effectiveness of behavioural interventions than are traditional group comparison research designs.

Although early experimental psychology was often concerned with the careful investigation of individuals, the accepted method of research soon changed to using larger sample sizes. One of the main reasons for this was the development of more sophisticated statistical methods which permitted the examination of interrelationships between variables without the need for experimental manipulation. There was also a dissatisfaction with the absence of adequate controls within individual research. This led to the emergence of the basic control-group design, which soon became the accepted method of psychological research: one group, which were exposed to the experimental condition(s), was compared with another group (a control group), which were not. Statistical tests were then used to determine whether the experimental condition produced an effect; i.e. whether it was statistically significant according to preselected levels of 'confidence' (probability levels). It was argued that larger sample experiments were more 'powerful' — i.e. better able to detect an experimental effect; as well as providing greater evidence for the generality of an observed relationship. If the relationship between the independent and dependent variables was demonstrated across a large number of subjects, this meant that the results were not idiosyncratic. This approach to psychological research soon became the accepted 'standard', and although the methodology has become increasingly sophisticated in terms of the number of design options and statistical techniques, the basic rules of between-groups research remain the same today.

The history of individual case research within clinical psychology is somewhat different. Despite the influence from experimental psychology, many researchers continued to see the value of single-case research as a means of discovering vital information about the uniqueness of the individual, often submerged in group research. For example, Allport (1961) recommended the intensive study of the individual (which he termed the *idiographic approach*) as a supplement to the study of groups (which he called the *nomothetic approach*). Similarly, major developments in the theory and practice of several therapeutic approaches, such as psychodynamic therapy, have stemmed from the intensive study of the individual (e.g. Freud, 1933; Breuer and Freud, 1957). Even so, between-group designs became the dominant approach in clinical research, and despite their obvious limitations in this context are still widely used in current research.

In contrast, current single-case designs have emerged from specific research areas within psychology. This can be traced to the work of Skinner and the research on *operant conditioning*. He was concerned with studying the behaviour of individual organisms and determining the antecedent and consequent events that influenced behaviour. There was, and continues to be, a close relationship between the theoretical account of operant behaviour and the methodological approach towards experimentation and data evaluation — referred to as the *experimental analysis of behaviour* (cf. Sidman, 1960). Skinner focused on animal behaviour, and primarily on the arrangement of consequences that followed behaviour and influenced subsequent performance. This research led to a set of relationships or principles that described the processes of behaviour (such as reinforcement, punishment, extinction, etc.) that distinguished operant conditioning and then radical behaviourism as a distinct theoretical position (e.g. Skinner, 1938, 1953).

The experimental analysis of behaviour consists of several distinct characteristics which are integral to single-case research designs. First, there is a concern with studying the frequency of behaviour because it presents a continuous measure of behaviour, provides orderly data, and reflects immediate changes as a function of changing environmental conditions. Second, only a few subjects are involved in a given experiment, allowing for the clear observation of lawful behavioural processes in individual organisms which might be submerged in averaging performance across several subjects, as is usually done in group research. Third, because of the lawfulness of behaviour and the nature of the data from continuous frequency measures, it permits direct observation of the effects of various manipulations upon a subject's behaviour.

From this early animal research, interest developed in applying the principles of operant conditioning to human behaviour; although most of the initial studies were primarily of methodological interest. Their concern was to demonstrate the usefulness of the operant approach in studying human behaviour, and discover whether the principles derived from animal research could be applied to humans. The research by Bijou (1955, 1957) and Lindsley (1956, 1960) are examples of this approach. Incidentally, subsequent research on human operant behaviour has demonstrated that, while there are some similarities between the behaviour of humans and lower organisms, there are some important and critical differences which can be attributed to the presence of verbal behaviour in humans, and the special properties these behaviours possess (see Lowe, 1979, for a review).

The therapeutic potential of operant conditioning was soon recognised by many researchers (e.g. Lindsley, 1960, noted the reduction of symptoms among psychotic patients during experimental sessions), and the focus shifted in many studies to include 'clinically relevant' behaviours (Ayllon and Michael, 1959; Ayllon, 1963). For example, Ayllon and Michael (1959) used an extinction procedure to reduce delusional talk in a psychotic patient. Similarly, Ayllon (1963) used operant principles in an attempt to change 'problem' behaviours such as violence, with several long-term psychiatric patients. Ayllon and Azrin's research on token economy programmes (TEPs) stemmed directly from these early studies, and marks the first full application of operant principles with therapeutic change as the primary aim of the programme (Ayllon and Azrin, 1968). By the late 1960s the extension of the experimental analysis of behaviour to applied areas was recognised formally as *applied behaviour analysis* (Baer, Wolf and Risley, 1968). Since then there has been considerable research on the therapeutic utility of behaviour analysis, and it is currently one of the major forms of intervention with many clinical 'problems'.

Although the history of operant conditioning and the development of single-case research designs are intertwined, the methodology has been extended beyond the conceptual framework and can be evaluated separately as a useful approach to applied and experimental research (see Kazdin, 1982a).

5.2 TOKEN ECONOMY PROGRAMMES

Over the past two decades the most widespread application of behavioural principles and methods in psychiatric hospitals has been in the form of token economy programmes (TEPs). Typically, there are three basic components to a TEP: first, a series of target behaviours specific to the particular subject group; second, a variety of back-up reinforcers; and third, tokens which the subjects 'earn' for correct performance of the target behaviours and which they may exchange according to a set of 'values' for items from the list of back-up reinforcers.

The use of TEPs has not been restricted to patients in psychiatric hospitals; since the early research conducted by Ayllon and Azrin (1968) TEPs have been successfully applied with a wide variety of clinical and non-clinical subject populations and in a variety of different settings (see Kazdin, 1977a and 1982b for reviews).

Like many forms of 'treatment' in psychiatry, the fortunes of TEPs have risen and fallen over the past few years. Kazdin, in his 1977 book *The Token Economy*, cites hundreds of research reports on the use of TEPs. Similarly, Baker, Hall, Hutchinson and Bridge, writing in 1977, claimed that 'the token economy is becoming an accepted clinical procedure for the rehabilitation of chronic psychiatric patients' (p. 381). However, since this time the flow of reports has significantly decreased, and currently only a trickle seem to appear in the literature. Of course, this does not mean that TEPs are no longer used to any great extent in a purely clinical manner, although even here there appears to be a similar decline. For example, in Watts and Bennett's important *Theory and Practice of Psychiatric Rehabilitation* (1983), there are only four references to TEPs, and these seem to occupy no more than four pages in total.

So what has happened to cause this change? It must be remembered that most of the early applications of TEPs in psychiatric hospitals were with groups of long-stay residents who typically, for various reasons, had similar skills deficits. It was reasonably straightforward, therefore, to set up a TEP: the target behaviours were usually the same for the whole group, and the items used as back-up reinforcers were powerful and relatively easy to control due to the institutional nature of the setting. Indeed, much of the early research was concerned with exploring the parameters of TEPs in such restricted environments (see Kazdin, 1977a). Since then there has been a marked change in both Britain and the USA in policy towards services for the chronic mentally ill. There are fewer long-stay residents in our psychiatric hospitals due both to successful rehabilitation/resettlement programmes and changed discharge policies. Similarly, the gradual establishment of appropriate community support services has led to a reduction in the number of chronic mentally ill becoming long-stay hospitalised patients. There are, however, a small but significant number of 'new long-stay' patients who seem to defy most current treatment practices — including behavioural interventions. Despite attempts to adapt TEPs to this changed service pattern; for example by individualising the target behaviours and token contingencies, comparatively few 'patients' live in settings where it would be either feasible or desirable to establish a TEP.

Over the past few years there has also been a growing concern with the ethics of TEPs. Many of the practices used in the early programmes, especially the selection and control of back-up reinforcers, were challenged, sometimes legally, and judged to be a contravention of some basic rights and/or undesirable. This has inevitably, although not necessarily (see later), led to a decline in the use of many behavioural interventions, especially TEPs.

Despite these changes, behavioural methods are still frequently used with chronic mentally ill people, although their use tends to be more selective, specific and with the consent of the individual concerned. It is perhaps even more important, therefore, to examine how behavioural interventions might be applied and suitably evaluated. In the remainder of this chapter I will be concerned with these methods of evaluation, and will describe in some detail an example drawn from a TEP. Although their use has declined, the methods used in evaluating TEPs and the issues these raise are also true for any behavioural interventions applied to chronic mentally ill people.

In token economy research two variations of the single-case design have been most commonly used. First, the ABAB design (e.g. Ayllon and Azrin, 1968): this examines the effect of an intervention by alternating the baseline condition (A) when no treatment is in effect, with the intervention condition (B). The effects of the intervention are clear if subjects' performance improves during the first intervention phase, reverts to, or approaches the original baseline levels when treatment is withdrawn; and improves when treatment is reinstated, etc. While being an effective research design, it is not without its limitations. The main drawback with the ABAB design is that it requires a 'reversal' of any behaviour change before valid conclusions can be reached about the effects of the intervention. This may not pose problems in many experimental situations but does cause difficulties in most clinical studies. More often than not, if a treatment is effective, it is therapeutically undesirable that there should be a reversal of the effect. Second, a design which avoids this problem is the multiple-baseline design. In this, baseline data are collected for two or more behaviours. Once performance has stabilised for all the behaviours, the intervention is applied to the first behaviour. If this behaviour changes but the others remain at their baseline levels, it suggests that the intervention was probably responsible for the change. Further evidence for the effectiveness of the intervention is gained if, when it is now applied to the second behaviour (as well as the first), this changes but the others continue to remain at their baseline levels. This procedure continues until the intervention has been introduced for all the behaviours. An example of the use of this design in TEP research is given in Nelson and Cone (1979). Of course, this design also has its limitations; for example, changes in one behaviour following the application of the treatment may produce changes in non-treated behaviours, or the treatment may have more of an effect on certain behaviours but not others. There is also the distinct possibility that the 'last' behaviour to be treated may be affected by extraneous factors, due to the delay before the treatment is introduced. Finally, treatment has to be withheld, often for lengthy periods, before being introduced for some behaviours, and this may not always be clinically desirable.

Therefore, while there are limitations to the multiple baseline design, these are relatively minor compared to the reversal problem described for ABAB designs, and this makes it the most appropriate type of research design for evaluating behavioural interventions (although see later for a useful application of an ABAB design).

(a) Behavioural targets/goals

The most important aspect of any behavioural intervention is the specification of the target behaviours or goals. Data are collected for these during the baseline and intervention phases, and given that the effectiveness of the intervention is determined through observing changes in the frequencies of these behaviours, then it is obvious that a great deal of precision is needed in specifying the target behaviours. They must be defined in ways which make observation and recording easy. This is usually achieved by *operationally defining* each behaviour; that is, describing the behaviour according to its specific components or its physical products. Either way, the description must allow the observer(s) to be able clearly, and with a high degree of agreement, to determine when the subject is performing the target behaviour, or when the appropriate physical changes have taken place. Ayllon and Azrin (1968) outline a number of 'rules' to follow in describing target behaviours, which are commendable in their breadth and clarity.

For example, if the target behaviours in a TEP include attempts to improve patients' self-help skills, it is not enough merely to state that one wishes for improvements in these skills, such as 'to increase patients' washing skills'. Instead, 'washing' has to be divided into its component skills, and decisions taken whether to record the performance of each component or their physical products. The following example is taken from a TEP the author was involved in. Washing was included as one of the target behaviours and it had been decided, through discussions with the staff, to record the products of this behaviour. The 'scoring' criteria were:

Each resident is encouraged to wash twice daily, once in the morning before breakfast has finished and once in the evening before retiring to bed. On both occasions the ward staff should observe the resident washing herself.

Token value 3 per item on both occasions if correct

(i) Hands, face and hair
√ = Hands and face have been washed and are thoroughly clean. Hair has been brushed or combed.
× = Hands and face have not been washed or not washed thoroughly. Resident has to be prompted to repeat process.

(ii) Teeth
√ = Resident is observed to have brushed her teeth or dentures. If resident has not teeth, rinses mouth out with water.
× = Resident does not brush teeth or dentures, or has not rinsed out mouth.

Even when detail such as this is included, there are inevitably some remaining 'grey' areas. In the above example, what is meant by 'clean'? Given that there is no 'right' or 'wrong' way to define washing, the exact definition of this skill must depend to a large extent on the consensus view of the staff administering the programme. Of course, this raises many important issues such as staff training and observer drift (cf. Kazdin, 1982b) etc., which are beyond the scope of this chapter.

In summary, the success of any attempt to evaluate a behavioural intervention depends almost entirely upon clearly defining the behaviours one is concerned with changing.

(b) Selection of target behaviours

Obviously, the target behaviours need to be clinically relevant to the individual or group subjected to the intervention. Yet it is surprising how many programmes, especially group-based ones, include target behaviours which some of the subjects can actually perform quite appropriately. More importantly, however, clinically relevant behaviours have a greater chance of maintaining once the intervention has been withdrawn (Kazdin, 1977a). Therefore, care needs to be taken over this selection process.

Most TEPs with long-term psychiatric patients have been

concerned with increasing the frequency of a range of adaptive behaviours, such as self-help, domestic, and social skills. Typically, this first involves some process of assessment; either by observation and interview, or through the use of some more structured means. There are several structured skills assessments available for use with long-term psychiatric patients (e.g. Barker, 1978; Hall and Baker, 1983). For example, the Everyday Living Skills Inventory (ELSI) devised by Barker (1978) includes 88 separate skills divided into categories such as communication, orientation, domestic, social skills, etc. Performance of each skill is assessed by matching an individual's present ability against one of six alternative descriptions. These are graded from either not performing the particular skill at all, or not having the opportunity to do so, through to independent performance. The outcome of this assessment is then neatly converted to a pictorial representation of the skill (in the form of a logo) which is shaded in according to the level of performance achieved.

Whichever method is used to identify either adaptive skills or problem behaviours, it forms the basis for specifying the target behaviours for an individual or group, as outlined above; and the task of collecting baseline data can begin.

(c) Measuring change

The system of measurement most commonly associated with behavioural interventions is direct observation (see Kazdin, 1982a for a fuller discussion). This comprises several strategies, each designed to measure changes in behaviour by directly observing and recording whether or not certain behaviours are occurring. For example, the frequency of a certain behaviour can be determined either by recording every instance of that behaviour, or by taking a number of discrete samples of the subject's general behaviour over a period of time (time-sampling), and then calculating the relative frequencies with which certain behaviours occurred. The type of direct observational method used is often determined by factors such as the absolute frequency of the behaviour under consideration (i.e. does it occur once per day or 100 times?), and the physical and administrative constraints upon the ability of the staff/researchers to observe the behaviours. Although labour-intensive and time-consuming, direct observation is the most reliable and effective means of evaluating any behavioural intervention.

In contrast, another method which has been widely used to measure change in patients' behaviour on a token economy (in Britain at least) is the rating scale. Typically, these consist of a number of items relating to certain aspects of the subjects' behaviour. The items are, by the very nature of a rating scale, usually preselected, and while they are generally applicable to the subject population of the study, rarely are they specific to any one individual. In completing a rating scale the rater is required to 'place' the subject at some point on a predetermined scale for each of the items. For example, a rater might be required to rate the frequency of a certain behaviour on a four-point scale ranging from 'never' through to 'very often'. Rating scales are usually completed at fixed intervals, such as daily, weekly or monthly.

Although a full discussion of the relative merits of rating scales is beyond the scope of this chapter, Hall (1980) in an excellent review examined 29 published ward behaviour rating scales for use with long-stay patients. Each was evaluated according to a number of criteria dealing with aspects of scale construction and validity, etc. Only four of the 29 scales reviewed satisfied even Hall's subset of five minimal criteria of acceptability. These were the two Wing Ward Behaviour Rating Scales (Wing, 1960, 1961); the Psychotic In-patient Profile (Lorr and Vestre, 1969); and the Missouri In-patient Behaviour Scale (Missouri Medical School, 1974).

While rating scales and direct observational methods raise somewhat different methodological issues about the measurement and recording of behaviour, they also share some in common. For example, the selection and training of observers/raters, the problem of inter-rater/observer agreement and the issue of observer bias (see Kazdin, 1977b for a discussion of factors influencing direct observational methods). Both approaches have their particular advantages and disadvantages. For example, Baker *et al.* (1977) have argued that the direct observation methods typically associated with behavioural interventions are limited. 'The usual behavioural approach has been to assess accurately specific items of "target behaviour" such as bed making, social interaction and shaving; but this approach often fails to assess concurrently other important areas of patient's functioning' (p. 382). However, this might be more a criticism of the application of direct observational methods rather than of the methodology itself. Any application should monitor the effects of an intervention on more than a few specific target behaviours. There is an obvious need to observe for changes in other, non-target, behaviours, as this allows for any generalisation of change to be detected as well as any undesirable changes in other behaviours.

A major limitation of rating scales is that the ratings are often completed at times other than when the patient(s) is engaged in the behaviour(s) which is being rated. Moreover, it is arguable that a rating scale is as much a measure of the observer's own behaviour and memory as it is of the patient's behaviour. The former may not always reflect the latter. Direct observation, on the other hand, requires the observer to record a patient's behaviour as and when it occurs by comparing it to a predetermined set of criteria.

A further advantage of direct observation is that the observer is continuously monitoring the effectiveness of the reinforcement contingencies in operation, and this can act as prompt to the observer to maintain consistent and regular delivery of the prescribed contingencies. This close 'contact' with the patient's behaviour might be a subtle yet important factor in the maintenance of any behavioural intervention. For example one of the contingencies in a TEP might be aimed at increasing patients' appropriate meal-time behaviour. Observing and recording patients' performance of these behaviours on each occasion, that is, three times each day, increases the likelihood that correct performances of these target behaviours are appropriately reinforced, as well as reducing the possibility that staff will 'miss' these opportunities. Direct observation methods, compared with rating scales, might also be useful therefore as a means of monitoring staff performance.

In summary, although direct observation is time-consuming it provides the most powerful method for evaluating any behavioural intervention, and has the advantage of being in close accord with the single-case methodology most commonly used in this research.

5.3 A CASE STUDY

The following illustration is drawn from a larger research

programme on token economy programmes in which the author was involved. This had been established in 1975 to meet the needs of a group of female long-stay patients at a large rural psychiatric hospital, many of whom would now be described as 'new' or 'young' long-stay. In addition to having vast deficits in most aspects of self-help and social skills, many displayed a variety of bizarre and psychotic behaviours. They had been 'collected' onto the ward in question because of their aggression and violence, and this had led not only to the ward being impoverished both in its material and social conditions but it also was continuously locked. In all respects, therefore, these patients were a deprived, disadvantaged and problematic group.

The initial aims of the TEP were to establish specific self-help, domestic and social skills common to the whole group. These included self-help skills such as washing, dressing appropriately, bathing; domestic skills such as bed-making, washing up, doing routine chores on the ward; and simple social skills such as joining in games and discussion groups. The patients were able to 'earn' specified numbers of tokens for each particular skill, which they were able to exchange for a variety of back-up reinforcers ranging from consumables through to items such as outings from the hospital. In many ways the programme was similar to most other TEPs with long-stay patients. Following the early success of the programme in bringing about some positive changes in many of the target behaviours, it was decided to investigate further two aspects of TEPs which had been generally overlooked.

First, most research on TEPs had looked at relatively short-term interventions; that is, weeks or months rather than years — there was little data on the long-term effects of a TEP (Rybolt, 1975; Paul and Lentz, 1977). In one study we (Woods, Higson and Tannahill, 1984) investigated changes in patients' performance of the target behaviours over a 5-year period. The main findings of this study were that some patients quickly responded to the token contingencies, and maintained these improvements once the contingencies had been removed. Using the definition outlined by Cullen, Hattersley and Tennant (1977) the programme had a truly *therapeutic* effect for these patients. An equal number of patients, however, responded relatively slowly, with positive changes in their behaviour only occurring in some instances after years of exposure to the programme contingencies. Moreover, these changes were fragile and frequently

107

reversed when the contingencies were removed. The programme could therefore be described as having a *prosthetic* effect in maintaining improvements in the behaviours of these patients (Cullen *et al.*, 1977). One conclusion of this study was that the phenomenon of subjects who are supposedly unresponsive to token contingencies (Kazdin, 1972), might be a consequence of the relatively short period of exposure to the contingencies reported in many studies, rather than to any actual lack of responsiveness. This study also highlighted the need to build into a TEP practices and procedures to maintain the programme itself (cf. Hall and Baker, 1973).

The second main aim of the research programme was to investigate the potential of a TEP in bringing about changes in patients' symptomatic behaviours. While there was some evidence that TEPs aimed at improving self-help skills sometimes also produced positive changes in symptomatic behaviours (e.g. Gripp and Magaro, 1974; Grzesiak and Locke, 1975; Schwartz and Bellack, 1975), these were coincidental when they occurred, and there were a number of studies in which such effects had not been found (see Bridge, 1974; for a review). The only studies which had demonstrated the effectiveness of token contingencies in producing positive changes in symptomatic behaviours were characterised by having been carried out in 'special' sessions away from the ward, and with poor evidence for generalisation of any positive changes from these sessions to other settings. No studies had successfully demonstrated positive changes in patients' symptomatic behaviours as a result of incorporating symptom-relevant targets into a ward-based programme.

In our study we investigated this using a single-subject multiple baseline research design (Tannahill and Higson, 1985). The symptomatic behaviours of seven patients were detailed and operationally defined in such a manner that the nursing staff were able directly to observe and record the particular symptomatic behaviours, or their overt components at least, for each of the seven patients. Specific token contingencies were then introduced for each of the symptomatic behaviours for each patient. The effects of these interventions were evaluated using both direct observation of any behavioural changes which occurred, and a standardised psychiatric rating scale — the Present State Examination (PSE) (Wing, Cooper and Sartorius, 1974). The PSE consists of 140 items, mostly in the form of questions, concerned with assessing a patient's general psychiatric state. The answers are rated according to presence/absence and severity, and then computed to provide a profile of a patient's main symptoms and syndromes. These were completed during the baseline phase and after the last of the interventions for each patient. The behavioural observations were continued for a further 6 months, at the end of which a third PSE was carried out.

The main outcome of this study was that the token contingencies *did* produce positive changes in patients' symptomatic behaviours when these were incorporated as targets in a ward-based TEP. There was also a high degree of correlation between the behavioural observations and the results of the PSE in each case. Furthermore, these positive changes were maintained to a large extent for the 6 months after the interventions were terminated. However, not all the symptomatic behaviours improved for any one patient, nor the same symptomatic behaviours for different patients. The reasons for this variability are outlined in Tannahill and Higson (1985), although the most likely explanation is that, even with the sensitive research design we employed, it failed to reflect the complex and possibly unique relationships which exist between symptomatic behaviours and their covert and overt determinants for each patient.

During the period between the establishment of the TEP and the second study outlined above, a growing concern was expressed, particularly by the nursing staff, about the items used as back-up reinforcers in the programme — specifically the use of meals in this way. Although this could have been construed exclusively as an ethical question we decided to carry out a simple piece of evaluative research. Our experimental question, therefore, was: is it necessary to use meals as a back-up reinforcer to maintain subjects' performance of a range of target behaviours in a TEP? Given that meals had been used in this way since the inception of the TEP it was decided to examine the effects of introducing them on a non-contingent basis.

Ayllon (1963) and Ayllon and Houghton (1962) demonstrated that food could function as a powerful reinforcer for the behaviour of hospitalised psychotic patients and, not surprisingly, many of the early TEPs included access to meals as a token-contingent back-up event (e.g. Schaefer and Martin, 1969). Since then many TEPs have included meals as a back-up event (Kazdin, 1977a) despite their ethical dubiousness. However in an institutional environment which offers few alternatives, it is almost inevitable that food will be one of the few potential reinforcers available. It is possible to understand, therefore, why so many TEPs have used meals in this way.

A wide variety of back-up events are usually incorporated into a TEP to maximise the 'value' of tokens and consequently the likelihood that clients will perform behaviours that earn them. In TEPs with hospitalised psychiatric patients, back-up events have often included such basic items as access to a bedroom, clothes, meals, or — more commonly — improvements in each of these over very minimal facilities (Kazdin, 1977a). Additional back-up events may include privileges, 'luxury' items, or other consumables.

This practice of re-scheduling a patient's access to these amenities has occasionally led to conflict of interests between administrators of the programme, who regard it as justified — as a means to establish desirable behaviour in their clients — and other members of society (including patients themselves), who regard these practices as unethical and a contravention of basic rights. In the USA these conflicts have occasionally been brought before the courts (Wexler, 1973, 1975; Kazdin, 1977a). An example of such a case was that of Wyatt v. Stickney (1972), the main outcome of which was a court decision that a hospitalised psychiatric patient has a *constitutional right* of access to a variety of events; for example, a comfortable bed, a wardrobe for clothing, a chair, nutritionally balanced meals, to receive visitors, to wear his/her own clothes, to attend religious services, to exercise several times weekly, to be outdoors regularly and frequently, to interact socially with the opposite sex, and to have a television in the day-room. Other legal cases in the USA have also concluded that unless a patient gives prior *informed consent*, he/she must have free access to basic rights and amenities, as decided by the courts. Similar cases or court rulings outlining an individual's rights have not been recorded in Britain, possibly due to the absence of a written constitution. However, a number of public inquiries have taken place into those programmes and procedures which have been seen as contravening basic rights and the general ethical standards of society (e.g. Napsbury Report; HMSO, 1973).

These have led to concern being expressed by a number of

individuals and groups about the ethics of behavioural programmes, and a government working party has reported upon ethical guidelines for behavioural treatment programmes (HMSO, 1980). However, this only has the status of an advisory document, and has no statutory mandate. What is lacking in this debate, however, is empirical evidence that to facilitate behaviour change it is *necessary* to restrict a client's access to certain basic amenities.

(a) Method

Subjects

Nine of the residents of the TEP ward served as subjects in this study. The remaining seven residents were also included but, for a variety of reasons, the data obtained from them were not included. Some were on individual programmes which were changed, while others either joined or left the ward during the course of the study. All nine subjects had been resident on the ward for at least 1 year prior to the commencement of the study; all were diagnosed as having chronic schizophrenia and were in receipt of maintenance doses of medication, which remained unchanged throughout the period of the study.

Procedure

Phase 1 — Contingent meals (1)   During the 12-week period preceding the experimental phase the nursing staff administered the TEP in the normal manner. They continued directly to observe and record the subjects' performance of the self-help, domestic and social skills specified as targets for all the residents on the TEP. Tokens were presented to the subjects for correct performance of these skills as before, who in turn could use them to purchase items from a list of 22 back-up reinforcing events, including meals. The 'cost' of purchasing all meals for any one day represented approximately 20 per cent of their token 'earning' potential for that day. The subjects were also able to purchase part-meals.

Throughout this phase the staff made no references to the patients about the impending introduction of non-contingent meals.

Phase 2 — Free meals (1)   The first experimental condition lasted for 12 weeks. During this phase all meals were provided on a non-contingent basis; i.e. were freely available to all the patients on the ward. At the beginning the nursing staff informed the patients that they would no longer be required to pay for meals with tokens, and that all meals were to be provided 'free of charge'. No extra encouragement was given to attend at meal times, nor did the staff repeatedly remind the patients that they were no longer required to 'pay' with tokens. In every other respect the administration of the TEP was unchanged.

Phase 3 — Contingent meals (2)   The conditions were reversed so that the patients were once again required to 'pay' for their meals (as in phase 1). The nursing staff informed all the patients that the period of free meals had now ended, and that they would once again have to 'pay'; this phase continued for 12 weeks.

Phase 4 — Free meals (2)   The conditions described in phase 2 were reinstated for a 12-week period.

Results

For each subject, data were collected over the four phases on: (i) the number of meals eaten; (ii) their performance of the target behaviours; and (iii) the pattern of token spending.

The number of meals eaten is shown in Figure 5.1. Each point represents the median percentage of meals eaten each week by the nine subjects, calculated on the basis of the number eaten, including half-meals, out of a possible weekly maximum of 21. During the two free meals phases of the study the subjects were eating slightly more meals each week than in the contingent meals phases.

These data, together with those collected for the self-help, domestic and social skills, were subjected to two types of statistical analysis. First, analyses of variance were carried out to determine whether there was any treatment effect following the introduction of free meals. The only significant effect was found for the number of meals eaten. Subjects' performance of the target behaviours was *not* affected by the introduction of free meals. The second analysis involved examining the same data for trends over the whole study, to determine whether the significant effect found for the number of meals eaten reflected

Figure 5.1: Proportion of meals eaten by the nine patients during the two experimental conditions

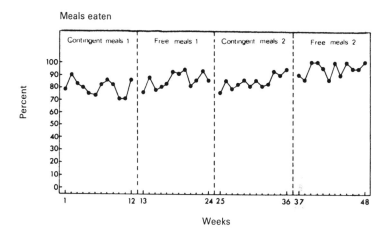

an underlying trend in the data rather than a treatment effect. This was carried out using the procedure outlined for time series data by Gottman, McFall and Barnett (1969). This confirmed that the increase in the number of meals eaten was not due to an underlying trend in the data, but was a real treatment effect following the introduction of free meals.

Figure 5.2 shows the median percentage of tokens spent each week on the three categories of back-up events: (i) meals, (ii) other consumables such as cigarettes, sweets, drinks; and (iii) other back-up reinforcers such as ward outings, etc. The introduction of free meals resulted in a large increase in the percentages of tokens spent by patients on other consumables, accounting for most of the tokens spent previously on meals. These returned to the previous levels when meals were once again scheduled as a back-up reinforcer, in phase 3. There were no systematic differences in the percentage of tokens spent on meals in the two contingent phases (1 and 3), and no systematic differences in the percentage of tokens spent on other back-up events in any of the four experimental phases. During the initial weeks of the first free meals phase (2), three out of the nine subjects were spending far fewer tokens than they had done in the previous weeks. This suggests that some of the subjects took longer to adjust their token spending pattern than others.

113

Figure 5.2: The proportion of tokens spent each week on meals, other consumables and other reinforcers

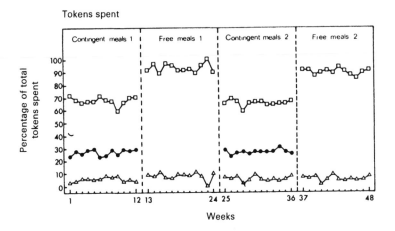

Key

● Meals
□ Other consumables
△ Other back-up events

However this effect was not general, and did not persist beyond the first few weeks; it did not occur in the second free meals phase (4).

(b) Discussion

Contrary to expectations, meals were not a critical back-up event in the present TEP. This was probably due to the fact that there was a wide range of other back-up events available within the programme, with sufficient 'demand' for them by the patients, so that when meals were made freely available they switched their token spending to other events. Interestingly, the pattern of spending changed in only one major respect — a large increase in the amount spent on other consumables such as cigarettes, drinks and sweets; but little change in spending on other back-up events such as trips off the ward. While the relative unimportance of meals solved one ethical dilemma, the observed increase in spending on cigarettes and sweets posed another equally contentious one.

The selection of back-up events in a token economy has, as Kazdin (1977a) points out, received little attention in research. Theoretically, *any* event could be used as a back-up reinforcer, if it could be demonstrated to have the effect of producing an increase in the probability or frequency of a subject's behaviour. One way to resolve the ethical dilemmas with regard to the selection of back-up reinforcers in a TEP would be to attempt to identify idiosyncratic and novel events which would function as reinforcers, and which are free of the more obvious ethical problems associated with food or cigarettes. Practices of this kind in *any* behavioural programme are in themselves desirable, and at the same time are likely to be more publicly acceptable on ethical grounds.

Both the actual results of this study and their wider implications were incorporated into the organisation of our TEP. The practice of using meals as a reinforcer was discontinued, with no apparent decline in the effectiveness of the programme. Also, a systematic review of the other back-up events was carried out, and over the next 3 years there was a deliberate and largely successful move away from using contentious items such as cigarettes and sweets as reinforcers. Instead, a wider variety of off-ward events were arranged, together with a system of 'weighting' the value of these events according to the expressed preferences of each individual.

In summary, the above piece of evaluative research, although relatively simple in its design and application, demonstrated how this approach could be used to answer a specific question about our use of behavioural methods in this context. Interestingly, following this study all staff involved with the programme showed an increased interest in applying similar research designs to evaluating other aspects of this 'service'.

5.4 CONCLUSION

In this chapter I have tried to highlight some of the issues involved in evaluating behavioural interventions, in particular TEPs, in psychiatric hospitals. Although there has been a decline in the use of token programmes with long-stay residents in these settings, this is more the result of changing service needs and patterns of care rather than a 'failure' in the methods themselves. Behavioural interventions, for example in the form of social skills training or individualised goal plans, are still extensively and successfully used with chronic mentally ill people in a variety of settings. As this chapter has, I hope, demonstrated, the methodological and research issues raised in evaluating TEPs are equally valid in considering methods for evaluating all other types of behavioural interventions in any setting.

Finally, it is important that all interventions or types of service are subjected to appropriate evaluations: there is no substitute for relevant data in reaching decisions about their efficacy.

REFERENCES

Allport, G.W. (1961) *Pattern and Growth in Personality*, Holt, Rinehart and Winston, New York

Ayllon, T. (1963) 'Intensive Treatment of Psychotic Behaviour by Stimulus Satiation and Food Reinforcement', *Behaviour Research and Therapy*, *1*, 53-61

Ayllon, T. and Azrin, N.H. (1968) *The Token Economy: A Motivational System for Therapy and Research*, Appleton-Century-Crofts, New York

Ayllon, T. and Houghton, E. (1962) 'Control of the Behaviour of Schizophrenic Patients by Food', *Journal of the Experimental Analysis of Behaviour*, *5*, 343-52

Ayllon, T. and Michael, J. (1959) 'The Psychiatric Nurse as a Behavioural Engineer', *Journal of the Experimental Analysis of Behaviour*, *5*, 323-34

Baer, D.M., Wolf, M.M. and Risley, T.R. (1968) 'Some Current Dimensions of Applied Behavior Analysis', *Journal of Applied Behavior Analysis*, *1*, 91-7

Baker, R., Hall, J.N., Hutchinson, K. and Bridge, G. (1977) 'Symptom Changes in Chronic Schizophrenic Patients on a Token Economy: A Controlled Experiment', *British Journal of Psychiatry*, *131*, 381-93

Barker, P. (1978) *Everyday Living Skills Inventory: ELSI*, Tayside Area Clinical Psychology Department, Dundee

Bijou, S.W. (1955) 'A Systematic Approach to an Experimental Analysis of Young Children', *Child Development*, *26*, 161-8

Bijou, S.W. (1957) 'Patterns of Reinforcement and Resistance to Extinction in Young Children', *Child Development*, *28*, 47-54.

Breuer, J. and Freud, S. (1957) *Studies in Hysteria*, Basic Books, New York

Bridge, G.W.K. (1974) 'Review of Token Economy Studies Using General Assessment Procedures', unpublished report, University of Leeds

Cullen, C.N., Hattersley, J. and Tennant, L. (1977) 'Behaviour Modification: Some Implications of a Radical Behaviourist View', *Bulletin of the British Psychological Society, 30*, 65-9

Freud, S. (1933) *New Introductory Lectures in Psychoanalysis*, Norton, New York

Gottman, J.M., McFall, R.M. and Barnett, J.T. (1969) 'Design and Analysis of Research Using Time Series', *Psychological Bulletin, 73*, 299-306

Gripp, R.F. and Magaro, P.A. (1974) 'Token Economy Programs in the Psychiatric Hospital: Review and Analysis', *Behaviour Research and Therapy, 12*, 205-28

Grzesiak, R.C. and Locke, B.J. (1975) 'Cognitive and Behavioral Correlates to Overt Behavioral Change with a Token Economy', *Journal of Consulting and Clinical Psychology, 43*, 272

Hall, J.N. (1980) 'Ward Rating Scales for Long-stay Patients: A Review', *Psychological Medicine, 10*, 277-88

Hall, J.N. and Baker, R. (1973) 'Token Economy Systems: Breakdown and Control', *Behaviour Research and Therapy, 11*, 253-63

Hall, J.N. and Baker, R. (1983) *REHAB*, Vine Publishing Co., Aberdeen

Hersen, M. and Barlow, D.H. (1976) *Single-Case Experimental Designs: Strategies for Studying Behavior Change*, Pergamon, New York

HMSO (1973) *Report of a Professional Investigation into Medical and Nursing Practices on Certain Wards at Napsbury Hospital, Near St. Albans*, HMSO, London

HMSO (1980) *Report of the Joint Working Party to Formulate Ethical Guidelines for the Conduct of Programmes of Behaviour Modification*, HMSO, London

Kazdin, A.E. (1972) 'Nonresponsiveness of Patients to Token Economies', *Behaviour Research and Therapy, 10*, 417-18

Kazdin, A.E. (1977a) *The Token Economy: A Review and Evaluation*, Plenum, New York

Kazdin, A.E. (1977b) 'Artefact, Bias, and Complexity of Assessment: The ABC's of Reliability', *Journal of Applied Behavior Analysis, 10*, 141-51

Kazdin, A.E. (1982a) *Single-case Research Designs: Methods for Clinical and Applied Settings*, Oxford University Press, New York

Kazdin, A.E. (1982b) 'The Token Economy: A Decade Later', *Journal of Applied Behavior Analysis, 15*, 431-45

Lindsley, O.R. (1956) 'Operant Conditioning Methods Applied to Research in Chronic Schizophrenia', *Psychiatric Research Reports, 5*, 118-39

Lindsley, O.R. (1960) 'Characteristics of the Behavior of Chronic Psychotics as Revealed by Free-operant Conditioning Methods', *Diseases of the Nervous System* (Monograph Supplement), *21*, 66-78

Lorr, M. and Vestre, N.D. (1969) 'The Psychotic In-patient Profile: A Nurse's Observation Scale', *Journal of Clinical Psychology, 25*, 137-40

Lowe, C.F. (1979) 'Determinants of Human Operant Behaviour', in M.D. Zeiler and P. Harzem (eds), *Advances in Analysis of*

Behaviour, Vol. I: Reinforcement and the Organisation of Behaviour, Wiley, Chichester

Missouri Institute of Psychiatry (1974) *Missouri Inpatient Behavior Scale (MIBS),* University of Missouri School, Missouri

Nelson, G.L. and Cone, J.D. (1979) 'Multiple-baseline Analysis of a Token Economy for Psychiatric Patients', *Journal of Applied Behavior Analysis, 12,* 369-74

Paul, G.L. and Lentz, R.J. (1977) *Psychosocial Treatment of Chronic Mental Patients,* Harvard University Press, Cambridge, Mass.

Rybolt, G.A. (1975) 'Token Reinforcement Therapy with Chronic Psychiatric Patients: A Three Year Evaluation', *Journal of Behavior Therapy and Experimental Psychiatry, 6,* 188-91

Schaefer, H. and Martin, P. (1969) *Behavioral Therapy,* McGraw-Hill, New York

Schwartz, J. and Bellack, A.S.A. (1975) 'A Comparison of a Token Economy with Standard Inpatient Treatment', *Journal of Consulting and Clinical Psychology, 43,* 107-8

Sidman, M. (1960) *Tactics of Scientific Research,* Basic Books, New York

Skinner, B.F. (1938) *The Behavior of Organisms,* Appleton-Century-Crofts, New York

Skinner, B.F. (1953) *Science and Human Behavior,* Free Press, New York

Tannahill, M.M. and Higson, P.J. (1985) *The Use of Behavioural Interventions in Changing the Symptomatic Behaviours of People who have Chronic Schizophrenia,* Final Report to the DHSS (Welsh Office)

Watts, F.N. and Bennett, D.H. (eds), (1983) *Theory and Practice of Psychiatric Rehabilitation,* Wiley, London

Wexler, D.B. (1973) 'Token and Taboo: Behavior Modification, Token Economies and the Law', *California Law Review, 61,* 81-109

Wexler, D.B. (1975) 'Reflections on the Legal Regulation of Behavior Modification in Institutional Settings', *Arizona Law Review, 17,* 132-43

Wing, J.K. (1960) 'The Measurement of Behaviour in Chronic Schizophrenia', *Acta Psychiatrica Scandinavica, 35,* 245-54

Wing, J.K. (1961) 'A Simple and Reliable Sub-classification of Chronic Schizophrenia', *Journal of Mental Science, 107,* 862-75

Wing, J.K., Cooper, J.E. and Sartorius, N. (1974) *Measurement and Classification of Psychiatric Symptoms: An Instructional Manual for the PSE and CATEGO Programme,* Cambridge University Press, Cambridge

Woods, P.A., Higson, P.J. and Tannahill, M.M. (1984) 'Token Economy Programmes with Chronic Psychotic Patients: The Importance of Direct Measurement and Objective Evaluation for Long-term Maintenance', *Behaviour Research and Therapy, 22,* 41-51

Wyatt *v.* Stickney. Supp. 373,344F. Supp 387 (M.D. Ala. 1972) affirmed sub. nom. Wyatt *v.* Alderbolt, 503F. 2d 1305 (5th Cir. 1974)

6

Evaluation in Clinical Psychology:
Outcome Evaluation of a Routine Clinical Psychology Service

Derek Milne

6.1 INTRODUCTION

The main aim of this chapter is to describe an outcome evaluation of a routine clinical psychology outpatient service. Subsidiary aims are to review the relevant research literature and to summarise some of the problems and research strategies contained in these reports.

While this chapter will probably be of most interest to other psychologists, it is hoped that the experimental approach outlined here will have much wider relevance, since it appears to address more general problems relating to evaluative research and clinical work. For one thing, this study was conducted under routine service conditions — that is without any special resources or deviation from the normal flow of clinical work. This meant that clients were an unselected succession of referrals to an existing service, with all the difficulties that this implies (Cowen, Lorion and Dorr, 1974).

A second and related point about such an evaluation is that although this kind of service has gone on for many years, very little research has actually been conducted in which the topic is *routine* work. What we do have in the literature are a number of studies of new service developments, such as the attachment of psychologists to general practitioner (GP) surgeries, and research studies with carefully selected clients. Marks (1985), for instance, reduced his 254 referrals to 150 by applying seven selection criteria. These included such considerations as the problem being likely to respond to therapy and the absence of severe depression. Similarly, Firth and Shapiro (1986) required that their clients cleared six selection hurdles, including a brief

119

problem history (less than 2 years) and that their medication had not changed in the past 3 months. By virtue of this selection process only about half of the referred patients were offered treatment in these two studies, and the proportions actually starting treatment were 36 per cent and 43 per cent, respectively. Moreover, these select few are clearly those most likely to benefit from therapy. In contrast, a 'routine' service will typically exclude very few people from therapy, which means that many people who are unlikely to benefit will receive help.

As a consequence, we create two quite different impressions of the utility of a given treatment and the relevance of research. It is no doubt as hard for practitioners to accept the results from 'special' research projects as it is for those who conduct them to take 'routine' evaluative research seriously. For example, a survey indicated that 40 per cent of mental health professionals thought that there was no research which was relevant to their practice (Cohen, 1976).

Despite the lack of relevant research, psychologists have advocated abandoning work with individual clients in community settings in favour of other strategies of service provision (e.g. Hawks, 1981). This is by no means a novel phenomenon, since other traditional practices have been criticised and abandoned as blind service alleys, before a relevant and systematic evaluation has taken place. A case in point is staff training, which has been treated as a 'dead duck' in terms of improving the quality of institutional care. However, more thorough-going evaluations have resurrected the contribution psychologists can make by training others to act as therapy mediators, as well as developing our understanding of organisational change (Milne, 1986).

These general points, therefore, provide a context and rationale for the present study: we need to study routine work, since this is often quite different from special research projects; and we can benefit from examining traditional practice since the findings may be surprising. Not least, we can adopt the 'practitioner–scientist' approach and seek to bridge the credibility gulf between the two traditionally separate groups.

6.2   A REVIEW OF RELATED EVALUATIONS

The bulk of outcome research in clinical psychology has been concerned with carefully selected clients and specific treatment approaches. Moreover, it has typically been conducted in special research settings, such as universities. Amongst other things, these factors are associated with brief interventions, student subjects, short follow-up periods and highly limited evaluations of client change (Agras and Berkowitz, 1980). The upshot of all this is a large literature yielding statistically rather than clinically significant findings. These differences drive a wedge between scientists and practitioners (Barlow, Hayes and Nelson, 1984). Thus although there is undoubtedly much for us to learn from 'refined' research work (e.g. regarding measurement) our focus in this review is restricted to routine or 'crude' research. This is exemplified by the recent work of psychologists in 'primary care'. This refers in practice to work in community clinics, health centres and GP surgeries, where the theme is to see clients during the early stages of their problems rather than during subsequent stages of care, as in the traditional area of rehabilitation. We will review this research briefly, in terms of the different kinds of evaluations that have occurred to date.

(a) Evaluating clients' needs

The initial research in primary care focused on the range and extent of problems that were relevant to clinical psychology and which were presented to GPs. The general background was provided by a large survey of 50 London practices by Shepherd, Cooper, Brown and Kalton (1966). This suggested that psychological problems had a total prevalence rate of 14 per cent, but that only 5 per cent of these clients were referred for specialist treatment.

Subsequent surveys focused on what services might be provided, to try and help more of these 14 per cent with problems. Davidson (1977), for one, surveyed GPs in London ($N = 76$) in order to establish the kinds of demands they would like to place on psychologists. Help in dealing with clients' sexual and marital problems was most often requested (57 per cent of GPs), closely followed by phobic disorders, addictive problems, obesity and obsessional–compulsive disorders. The surveyed GPs also requested assessment facilities (e.g. intellectual, vocational) and some teaching for themselves. McPherson and Feldman (1977) sat in on regular GP surgeries, with both GP and psychologist making independent ratings of the relevance of

121

psychological factors to a client's presenting problem. A sample of clients who were rated by the psychologist as either 'quite relevant' or 'highly relevant' on the psychological factors were then interviewed in more detail, in order to estimate the contribution a psychologist might make to their care. In this way it was judged that a psychologist could offer a useful clinical intervention in 8 per cent of the cases who consulted their GPs during the initial sitting-in phase.

(b) Evaluating treatment outcome

Evaluations of the contribution psychologists can make with such clients as those indicated above have taken a variety of forms. The initial studies relied on a simple judgement of improvement. Clark (1979), for instance, utilised a three-point scale, ranging from 'no improvement' through 'slight improvement' to 'great improvement'. The ratings were made jointly by psychologist and client in relation to predetermined definitions. Thus 'great improvement' was judged to have occurred if both of them regarded the client as free of symptoms and of personal difficulty. In this way 50 per cent of the treated clients were rated as 'greatly improved', 38 per cent as 'slightly improved', and the remaining 12 per cent as 'not improved'. Ives (1979) applied a similar rating scheme with a series of 185 clients, obtaining very similar outcomes to those above (i.e. 72 per cent improved). Ives also conducted 3-month and 1-year follow-up evaluations, finding indications from surgery visits and prescriptions that the clients had maintained their improvement.

The first controlled evaluation of outcome was reported by Earll and Kincey (1982). They assigned 50 consecutive referrals to either behaviour therapy with the psychologist or management by their GP. Also, unlike the foregoing studies, the effects of these forms of treatment were evaluated by published questionnaires rather than by *ad hoc* ratings. A further enhancement of the experimental design was the use of an independent assessor to judge the client's progress. However, no significant differences were found between the groups seen by the psychologist or the GPs on objective measures (prescriptions, consultations, use of hospitals) or on the questionnaires. In contrast, 85 per cent of the psychologists' clients perceived the therapy as either helping 'definitely' or 'to some extent', a finding corroborated by the independent assessor.

More recently Robson, France and Bland (1984) have reported a more careful outcome evaluation. A similar control group design to that of Earll and Kincey (1982) was adopted, but this time four subsequent assessments were conducted over a 1-year period. These were based on nine-point rating scales, covering the severity of the problem, effect on the client (both of which were judged by the GP and the client), and effect on the household (judged by a member of the household). Ten weeks were allowed for psychological treatment, after which an independent GP conducted a 'blind' assessment (i.e. unaware of the client's group membership), using the same rating scales of problem severity and effect on client. The results suggested that the group seen by the psychologist had significantly reduced 'problem severity', 'effect on household' and 'effect on sufferer' ratings at the time of their first three assessment periods (14, 22 and 34 weeks after therapy), as judged by both client and independent GP. But at a 1-year follow-up assessment the GP ratings for the group treated by the psychologist were not significantly better than those for the control group, although clients in the treated group still rated themselves as better off on the 'severity of problem' and 'effect on sufferer' scales. In summary, therefore, the involvement of a clinical psychologist seemed to accelerate the improvement of clients, but by the 1-year follow-up period the control group had also improved by a comparable degree, as rated by the independent GP. As far as the clients themselves were concerned, though, the treated ones continued to rate themselves as significantly more improved than did their counterparts. Robson *et al.* (1984) concluded that many problems were short-term and related to life transitions, but they considered that the intervention of a psychologist was nonetheless worthwhile.

(c) Evaluating economic outcome

In addition to the clinical outcomes just discussed, Robson *et al.* (1984) also evaluated some of the financial consequences of the work of the clinical psychologists in the health centre. They quantified visits to the GP and prescription costs, finding that the treated group reduced visits both during and after seeing the psychologist, and that there had been a similar saving on prescriptions. These statistically significant findings were calculated to be worth two sessions a week of a psychologist's time, in terms of the drug reductions alone.

In fact, economic evaluations were amongst the first type of assessments to be applied to the work of psychologists. Koch (1979), for instance, examined GP consultations and psychotropic drugs over a period of 1 year before and after treatment, reporting a 50 per cent reduction in prescriptions consequent on seeing the psychologist, as well as less demand on GP time. Ives (1979) reported an identical reduction in prescriptions and similar drop in GP consultations. However, a subsequent controlled study by Earll and Kincey (1982) found that although their patients received significantly less psychotropic medication by the end of treatment this was not maintained at a 7-month follow-up assessment.

A subsequent analysis by Freeman and Button (1984) shed some light on these discrepant findings. They reported that although patients who had seen the clinical psychologist showed marked reductions in both GP consultations and prescriptions, this simply reflected a general trend throughout the group practice. Furthermore, when they examined the records of all patients with at least one psychological problem over a 6-year period they found evidence of a 'worst-year' phenomenon, in which such problems had a natural history of crisis and remission. This led them to conclude that there is no benefit attendant upon seeing the psychologist. Their results also raise questions about the validity of follow-up data on a service, in the absence of comparative information about the general trends within a setting.

(d) Evaluating client satisfaction

As discussed in Chapter 1, outcome and other evaluations do not always correspond with the clients' rating of a service. A case in point was Freeman and Button's (1984) generally pessimistic conclusions regarding the value of individual therapy, which were tempered by the 'evident enthusiasm' (p. 379) of both clients and GPs for the clinical psychology service. Earll and Kincey (1982) also reported a high degree of client satisfaction: 45 per cent said that seeing a psychologist had 'definitely helped a great deal' and 40 per cent that it helped 'to some extent'. Only 18 per cent said that it had not helped at all. These findings were corroborated by an independent therapist's ratings of client satisfaction.

To some extent GPs are also clients who 'use' psychological services. It is therefore appropriate to assess their feelings about the service too. Jerrom, Simpson, Barber and Pemberton (1983) surveyed 50 GPs, finding very high levels of GP satisfaction: 98 per cent regarded the psychology service as a 'very useful' or 'useful' addition to primary care, and all GPs thought the service should be continued or expanded.

(e) Process evaluations

The foregoing evaluations consider either the 'input' to (e.g. client characteristics) or 'output' from a service (e.g. clinical change). What they omit to do is study the 'throughput' or process by which the outcomes are achieved. This is an understandable state of affairs in a relatively new service development, but it does not help us to clarify the possible reasons for clinical change. The strikingly similar findings mentioned above (about 70 per cent of clients improved) suggest that the psychologists were all equally effective. If this is true, it becomes particularly important to find out why, over and above the contribution of any 'non-specific' therapeutic effects. Yet the reports reviewed above are extremely vague and unforthcoming about therapists and their therapy process. Freeman and Button (1984) only refer to the psychologist providing 'individual therapy' (p. 379), with no clarification of even the general approach that was used. Earll and Kincey (1982) were more helpful, stating that: 'treatment was largely based upon a behavioural self-control model. Specific behavioural techniques were used wherever appropriate, following initial analysis of the problems' (p. 34). Koch (1979) went further, and cited examples of the techniques he used, including systematic desensitisation, modelling, response prevention and social skills training as part of a behavioural psychotherapy approach.

The possible variety in the actual treatments offered is underscored by Robson et al.'s (1984) account of their clinical psychologists. They were all, they report, 'behaviourally orientated, but otherwise their background, experience, and interests were sufficiently widespread to reflect the profession as a whole' (p. 1806). Since we know that different therapists can produce very different outcomes (Brooker and Wiggins, 1983) there is a pressing need to evaluate the effects of the therapist/therapy variables. Beck (1979) has produced a 'competency checklist' to facilitate such quantification with cognitive therapists, and in a related study to the one reported below we evaluated therapy and therapist by means of audio-tape recordings and client ratings of the therapy process (Milne and Castle, 1986).

It is perhaps worth noting that this general lack of attention to process or 'independent' variables is widespread in clinical psychology. Peterson, Homer and Wonderlich (1982), for example, surveyed articles in the behavioural literature and found that the majority did not assess the actual occurrence of the independent variable, and a sizeable minority did not even define it. As they pointed out, systematic research requires us to demonstrate a causal relationship between therapy and outcome.

6.3 AN OUTLINE OF THE PRESENT EVALUATION

The study we are about to consider was intended to evaluate the effects of a routine clinical psychology service on a series of unselected clients attending a National Health Service (NHS) clinic. The clinic was sited near the centre of Wakefield, a small city near Leeds in West Yorkshire, UK. It was used by a variety of community health services including chiropodists, health visitors and community physicians. The psychology service had been in operation from this base for several years beforehand.

A 1-year sample of consecutive referrals to this clinic was studied. The goal of the service was to help clients to understand and to develop self-control over their problematic symptoms. Specifically, I aimed to increase the clients' scores on our measure of 'active cognitive' and 'active behavioural' coping (CRQ) by a significant amount over baseline scores and to reduce their symptoms or 'strain' (GHQ) in the same way as a result of therapy.

During appointments clients were seen individually by the author, at that stage a senior-grade clinical psychologist working for the NHS. My qualification to practice was the Diploma in

Clinical Psychology, awarded by the British Psychological Society (BPS). I had been qualified for 5 years at the start of the study and had been in supervised training for 3 years prior to that period. My therapeutic orientation was behavioural.

A 'waiting list control group' design was employed, with repeated assessments being conducted over a 17-month period stretching from time of referral to 1 year after the client's first appointment. The measures used were self-report questionnaires and rating scales concerned with the clients' 'stress', 'coping' and 'strain', supplemented by ratings made by referring agents.

The main reason for selecting this combination of questionnaires was to try and determine the relationship between the clients' 'stress', 'coping' and 'strain' over the study period. This approach was used because the studies reviewed above had restricted themselves to simple ratings of 'strain', namely symptoms such as anxiety, depression, or more often simply of general psychological well-being. However, in therapy it is quite possible that factors other than the treatment may be responsible for client improvement. One such factor is reduced 'stress', by which we refer to problematic life experiences that require a reaction, as exemplified by such life events as getting married, changing jobs or moving house. In this sense a client may be reporting less strain after 3 months of therapy, but this may be attributable to other concurrent life changes, as suggested by Freeman and Button (1984). This then places an onus on us to assess a third factor, 'coping', which refers to the client's problem-solving efforts, as in seeking advice or taking action to alter the source of stress (Cohen and Lazarus, 1979). Taken together, assessments of these three factors can tell us much more about the effect of therapy than a simple measure of strain. For one thing, they may exclude the explanation of reduced stress mentioned above. But perhaps more significantly, they can tell us whether our therapy has had any effect on the client's coping, the main focus of our intervention, and the relationship of this to their reported strain. This analysis, therefore, provides a more comprehensive account of individual change and allows us to judge our contribution with more confidence than a simple assessment of strain. Table 6.2 indicates which questionnaires were used to assess stress, coping and strain. This kind of analytic framework has been discussed and endorsed by Cohen and Lazarus (1979) and Gottlieb

(1983). It appears to enjoy wide acceptance amongst psychologists for the kinds of reasons given above. We will refer to the stress–coping–strain framework as the 'coping cycle'.

6.4 CLIENTS

During the one calendar year studied, 35 clients on an existing waiting list were sent first appointments in order of referral. Of these, 25 participated in the evaluation, three did not attend their first appointment, four dropped out before treatment started and three were not suitable for treatment. The remainder of this report therefore concerns those 25 clients who were treated. A summary of some background factors and their characteristics is given in Table 6.1. It can be seen that the clients were referred equally by GPs and psychiatrists, both of whom retained an active involvement in their treatment. This is reflected in 65 per cent of the clients being on medication at the time of their first appointment, and by the relatively high frequency of GP attendances in the last year. The bulk of the clients were in non-professional employment, such as clerical workers (social class 3), agricultural workers (4) and labourers (5). The group were split almost exactly by sex, and the major reason for referral was anxiety. The mean age (35 years) and the problem duration (9 years) were very similar to those of the clients seen in the Marks (1985), and Durham and Turvey (1986) studies.

6.5 RESEARCH DESIGN AND ASSESSMENT PROCEDURE

Clients referred to the psychology service were sent an acknowledgement letter and asked to complete and return (in an enclosed stamped addressed envelope) a batch of questionnaires within a week of receiving our letter. These questionnaires were completed for a second time after the initial appointment, once we had explained the rationale for the procedure (namely, to assess problem areas and to evaluate the effect of our treatment).

During this first appointment we also outlined the emphasis we placed on 'self-control', the likely time scale and appointments we would require, answered any questions, and defined

Table 6.1: A breakdown of the clients' (*N* = 25) background information and characteristics, at the time of their first appointment. (Please note: several columns do not sum to 100% because clients experienced multiples of some variables, for example taking anxiolytic and antidepressant medication at the same time.)

Background information						Client characteristics				
Live alone (%)	Source of referral (%)	Client's estimate of problem duration (years)	Time since first contact with mental health services (years)	Disciplines involved (%)	Medication	Client's estimate of number of GP consultations in last 12 months	Age (years)	Social class (%)	Nature of problem identified in referral (%)	Sex
	GP Psychiatrist	Mean S.D.	Mean S.D.			Mean S.D.	Mean S.D.			
14%	56% 44%	8.6 6.01	4.8 4.4	GP 80%	Anxiolytic 50%	8.2 7.05	35.5 10.43	1: 12%	Generalised anxiety or tension 48%	48% female
				Psychiatrist 60%	Anti-depressants 45%			2: 9%	Depression 20%	52% male
				Community psychiatric nurse 10%	Hypnotics 15%			3: 35%	Specific phobia 12%	
				Social worker 5%	Major tranquillisers 5%			4: 26%	Obsessional compulsive disorder 12%	
					No medication 35%			5: 9%	Sexual dysfunction 8%	
								Unemployed 9%		

with them their presenting problem. Once defined, we usually added one or more specific symptomatic questionnaires to the original batch. There was a deliberate attempt to postpone any potentially therapeutic techniques until after this second assessment was completed.

All questionnaires were re-administered after 3 months of appointments or at the end of treatment, whichever came first. A 'follow-up' assessment was carried out 3 months after the end of treatment, whenever that occurred. In sum, therefore, we were employing a repeated-measures design in which clients were assessed four times — twice before and twice after treatment. This allowed us to regard the client's initial two as baselines for the subsequent two assessments. During the first post-therapy assessment we also requested ratings from the referring agents. A summary of the measures and their time of administration is given in Table 6.2.

6.6   THERAPY PROCEDURE AND DESCRIPTION

Following the introductory first appointment, clients were seen for approximately 30 minutes every week or two until it was jointly agreed that appointments could either stop or be much less frequent. A record was maintained of the duration of all appointments, to the nearest 5 minutes, together with a note of non-attendances and the total number of appointments. This information is summarised in Table 6.3. The table shows that clients were seen on average 13 times for 33 minutes per appointment. Each client averaged one non-attendance during this period.

The psychologist's general orientation was behavioural. In practice this entailed an initial period when appointments were concerned purely with assessing the presenting problem so as to arrive at a formulation, as described by Kanfer and Saslow (1969). To facilitate this phase clients were typically asked to maintain a 'diary' between appointments. This was based on a functional analysis of the problem, and asked them to record antecedents, the nature of the problem and its consequences. These records were then discussed in detail along with further examples elicited in interview. In a minority of cases the problems were also observed directly or described by friends or relatives. By means of this information an attempt was made to

Table 6.2: A description of the measures

Title of measure	Source	When it was administered	Description
1. Schedule of Recent Events (SRE)	Tennant and Andrews (1976)	At referral, first appointment and 3 months into treatment	This was the 'stress' measure, being a comprehensive life event inventory suitable for questionnaire administration. Events assessed include health, bereavement, family and social, friends and relatives, education, work, and financial and legal. There are 67 items and the client ticks those that have occurred in the last year. Each tick counts as 1.
2. Coping Responses Questionnaire (CRQ)	Billings and Moos (1981)	As measure 1	Our 'coping' assessment was a 19-item form covering three methods of coping ('active cognitive', 'active behavioural' and 'avoidance') and two coping foci ('problem' or 'emotion' focused coping). A five-point frequency rating was employed, as suggested by the authors. This ranged from 'almost never' to 'almost always', scored from 0 to 4.
3. General Health Health Questionnaire (GHQ)	Banks, Clegg et al. (1980)	At referral, first appointment, 3 months into treatment, and at 3-month follow-up	The GHQ was regarded as assessing 'strain'. We used a twelve-item short version, with questions covering such thing as the client's ability to concentrate, sleep or make decisions, as well as asking them whether they had been feeling depressed or under strain. Reply options ranged from 'not at all' to 'much more than usual' with corresponding scoring from 0 to 3.
4. Self-rating Forms	Specially developed by the author	Three months into treatment, and 3-month follow up	Clients rate how well they think they are generally, and how the particular problem is that they saw the psychologist about at the outset. Seven-point rating scales were used, going from 'very much worse' to 'very much better', scored from 6 to 0.
5. Referring Agent's Rating Forms	Specially developed by the author	Three months into treatment	Referring agents (i.e. psychiatrists and GPs) also made the general and particular problem ratings as above. In addition they were asked where they would have referred to had they not used a psychologist, how long they had known the client and, lastly, how they had formed an opinion about their rating
6. Service Evaluation Questionnaire (SEQ)	Specially developed by the author	Three months into treatment	This measure is a 20-item rating scale, covering the aims, content, procedure and outcomes of the clients' appointments. Each item was rated between 'strongly disagree' to 'strongly agree' on a seven-point scale. Clients were asked to complete the questionnaire anonymously, and were encouraged to add any other comments at the foot of the form.

Table 6.3: Details of client attendance at appointments

Number of appointments	Duration of appointments (minutes)	Non-attendance at appointments
Mean: 12.8	Mean: 32.6	Mean: 0.9 (per client)
Range: 5-27	Range: 15-70	Range: 0-5
Standard deviation: 6.22	Standard deviation: 10.16	Standard deviation 1.19
		Overall percentage of appointments not attended: 11%

clarify regularities between the problem, the client's environment and their coping methods. A simple illustration would be that a client experiencing panic attacks in association with possible difficulty in getting home (e.g. markets, buses, queues, etc.) reacts to these symptoms by rushing out of such situations and by avoiding them in future.

Once an initial formulation of the client's presenting problem had been achieved this then guided attempts to intervene and alter their coping cycle. In the case of the simple illustration above, this might involve developing the client's understanding of anxiety, highlighting the thoughts they are having about the anxiety symptoms, training them in progressive muscular relaxation and changing their escape and avoidance behaviour toward feared situations. To facilitate this learning process we supplied clients with a self-help manual on anxiety management (Milne and Linford, 1984). A similar approach was followed with other kinds of problems, broadly as described in case studies in such journals as *Behaviour Research and Therapy, Behavioural Psychotherapy, Behaviour Therapy*, and *Cognitive Therapy*.

More detailed breakdowns of the actual content and process of the therapy sessions were reported in another paper (Milne and Castle, 1986). These were based on a sample of transcribed audiotape recordings of therapy sessions with these clients, and on their evaluations of the content and process of therapy. Some of this information was presented in Chapter 2.

6.7 RESULTS

The main findings for the 25 treated clients are summarised in Table 6.4. This is a preliminary analysis and gives their scores on the first three measures listed in Table 6.2, being the ones concerned with stress (SRE), coping (CRQ) and strain (GHQ). The proportions of administered questionnaires that were completed and usable were 96, 94 and 98 per cent, respectively.

Table 6.4: A summary of the findings obtained from the three principal measures of stress (SRE), coping (CRQ) and strain (GHQ), presented as mean scores ($\bar{X}$) and standard deviations (S.D.)

Measure	At time of referral		After first appointment	Three months after first appointment
Schedule of Recent Events (SRE)				
$\bar{X}$	3.7		3.9	3.9
S.D.	1.91		2.1	2.8
Coping Responses Questionnaire (CRQ)				
$\bar{X}$	Cognitive	1.9	1.7	2.1
	Behavioural	1.7	1.5	1.9
	Avoidance	1.6	1.5	1.5
S.D.	Cognitive	0.72	0.82	0.78
	Behavioural	0.79	0.73	0.64
	Avoidance	0.8	0.75	0.81
General Health Questionnaire (GHQ)				
$\bar{X}$	22.2		19.5	8.9
S.D.	10.5		8.71	5.99

If we study the results from each measure in turn, we can see firstly that the client's stress (SRE) remained constant throughout the evaluation period. In support of this, no statistically significant differences were obtained between any two assessment phases. The figures (3.7, 3.9, 3.9) represent the mean number of events reported by clients, and do not take into account the nature of the events experienced. However, since it is always difficult to predict whether any given event (e.g. pregnancy) is a 'desirable' or an 'undesirable' event for an individual (Redfield and Stone, 1979), a simple frequency count level is preferred. This allows us to note significant alterations in potential stressors, and when these are not found, as here, we are inclined to exclude this variable from our explanation for any obtained changes in coping or strain.

The second main measure, the Coping Responses Questionnaire (CRQ), yielded similar findings to the SRE during the baseline periods: no statistically significant change in the overall score or in the three CRQ components (i.e. coping by 'active cognitive', 'active behavioural' and 'avoidance' methods) was found between first and second baseline assessments. There was then a marked but non-significant trend for the CRQ score to increase by the 3 months of therapy assessment, in relation to both sets of baseline findings.

In a second analysis, those 'improved' clients who had shown substantial changes in strain following therapy (defined as a GHQ score reduction of 50 per cent or more) were considered separately from the remainder of the clients. On the 'coping cycle' logic that these 'improved' patients ($N = 14$) must have developed their adaptive coping skills (i.e. 'active cognitive' and 'active behavioural'), it was predicted that these would increase significantly by the time of the third assessment. The same reasoning led to the corollory prediction, namely that the 'unimproved' clients ($N = 11$) would not show any such increase in coping skills. Both of these predictions were upheld ($p < 0.05$; Wilcoxon), suggesting that when therapy was most effective in alleviating strain it appeared to do so by increasing the clients' adaptive coping skills.

Table 6.4 shows that the mean General Health Questionnaire (GHQ) score declined substantially between the second baseline and the 3-month therapy assessment. This change was significant at the 5 per cent probability level (Wilcoxon statistic) in comparisons made between both baselines and their intervention phase. The less marked decrease obtained in GHQ scores between the first and second baseline assessments was not significant statistically. It suggests that the care the clients were receiving (principally medication) from their GPs and psychiatrists was not alleviating their strain during this 5-month period. A fourth assessment, conducted 3 months after therapy had stopped (the 'follow-up'), produced a GHQ score that was not statistically different from the previous evaluation. This finding indicated that the clients had maintained their improvements following the termination of therapy.

In addition to the statistically significant reduction in GHQ scores, there was a corresponding reduction in the number of psychiatric 'cases', as classified by the GHQ. The number of 'cases' in the sample during the first and second baseline assessments was 10 (53 per cent) and 9 (47 per cent) respectively. By the time the clients had received 3 months of treatment from the psychologist the number of cases had dropped to 2 (9 per cent). There were the same number of cases at the follow-up assessment. These results indicated that the change in strain was also significant when expressed in broad clinical terms.

The GHQ findings were corroborated by the results derived from specific questionnaires, also administered after the first interview and 3 months into therapy. Depending on the presenting problem, clients were asked to complete such measures as the Fear Questionnaire (FQ — Marks and Mathews, 1979), Beck's Depression Inventory (BDI — Beck, Clegg, Jackson *et al.*, 1961) or the Maudsley Obsessional Compulsive Inventory (MOCI — Hodgson and Rachman, 1977).

Clients reported a significant reduction in the symptoms and problematic behaviours presented in these questionnaires, with an overall drop from 56 per cent of items affirmed down to 23 per cent (Wilcoxon, $p < 0.05$).

The clients' self-ratings of the 'particular problem' and their 'general well-being' were combined to yield an overall mean score. After 3 months of treatment this was 2.3, representing a rating between 'a little better' and 'quite a lot better'. Unfortunately, referring agents' ratings at the same point in time were only received from 12 (48 per cent) of the GPs/psychiatrists. Their independent ratings, using the same scales as the clients, produced a mean score of 1.8, representing a slightly better impression of clinical outcome, namely one between 'quite a lot better' and 'very much better', the top of our scale.

Our final measure, the Service Evaluation Questionnaire (SEQ) indicated that consumer satisfaction was generally very favourable. The SEQ items are presented in Table 6.5, together with the number of clients selecting each rating between 'strongly disagree' and 'strongly agree'. In the table the two extreme points (0,1 and 5,6) were combined for summary purposes, giving a five-point scale.

In a second analysis these replies were classified according to four factors, being the 'aims', 'content', 'process' and 'outcomes' of appointments, following Wolf (1978). This produced mean satisfaction ratings of 71 per cent on the 'content' items, 86 per cent on the 'process' ones, 84 per cent for the aims of our appointments and 67 per cent for the clinical outcomes. (A score of 0 per cent would represent absolutely no client satisfaction.) The 'outcome' rating was therefore least satisfactory, suggesting that the clients would have liked to have got better understanding and coping skills from appointments and a greater reduction in their problems.

Amongst the individual items, Table 6.5 shows that clients very strongly agreed with the duration of appointments, saw the appointments as very satisfactorily conducted, and regarded the psychologist as competent. There was less agreement on whether the psychologist had bolstered their confidence, and on whether they would make use of the self-control skills covered in appointments.

6.8   DISCUSSION AND CONCLUSION

In terms of helping clients to feel better the results indicate that the clinical psychologist was more effective than the waiting list conditions. 'Strain', as measured by the GHQ, specific questionnaires and by independent ratings by referring agents, dropped significantly during the first 3-month therapy period. This was in contrast to little improvement during a prior 5-month period when clients were seen by their GP and/or psychiatrist and treated largely by medication. These findings were maintained at a 3-month follow-up assessment.

The obtained improvement did not seem to be due to systematic changes in the stressful life events encountered by clients, since the number of events remained constant during the evaluation period. This finding, and the baseline GHQ scores, suggest that these clients were not experiencing transitory, stress-induced strain as suggested by Robson *et al.* (1984) or Freeman and Button (1984). The implication is that this sample of clients *do* require and benefit from a therapeutic intervention, rather than improving either as stressors ease, via medication, or by some of the other variables present during waiting list conditions. Marks (1985), and Durham and Turvey (1986), also found little or no improvement amongst their comparably chronic group during waiting list conditions.

Table 6.5: A summary of the clients replies on the service evaluation questionnaire (18 (72%) clients completed the form)

	Strongly disagree	Mildly disagree	In-between or can't decide	Mildly agree	Strongly agree
1. The service helped me with my problem	0	1	4	1	12
2. I agreed with the aims of the service	0	0	3	1	14
3. The psychologist helped me to develop useful coping skills	0	1	4	2	11
4. The psychologist added to my understanding of my problem	1	0	3	3	11
5. The content of appointments could be improved	11	0	5	1	1
6. Appointments should be shorter	16	1	1	0	0
7. Self-control is an important topic to cover during appointments	1	2	4	2	9
8. The psychologist has helped me to become more confident	3	0	5	2	8
9. I expect to make considerable use of self-control skills (e.g. relaxation)	2	0	7	2	7
10. The psychologist was competent	0	0	3	0	15
11. Other people would approve of the psychologist's aims	0	0	6	0	12
12. I found it easy to understand the psychologist	0	0	1	1	16
13. Other people would approve of the way the psychologist worked	0	0	3	2	13
14. The appointments were conducted in a satisfactory manner	0	0	2	0	16
15. Too many irrelevant things were discussed	13	3	1	0	1
16. Not enough time was spent on assessing and understanding my problem	13	1	2	1	1
17. I felt comfortable with the psychologist	0	0	4	2	12
18. It would have been better to have spent more time developing my self-control	9	1	5	3	0
19. Generally, I agreed with the things which the psychologist was trying to achieve	0	0	3	1	14
20. Trying to understand my problem was a valuable exercise	0	0	5	1	12

Furthermore, the indication from our third main instrument, the Coping Responses Questionnaire (CRQ), was that therapy reduced strain by increasing adaptive coping skills, specifically the 'active cognitive' and 'active behavioural' methods of dealing with stress. This possibility was borne out by the significant increase in these two forms of coping only in the case of those clients who had improved clinically by a substantial amount. The remaining clients did not show any comparable change in coping, nor did either sample improve those skills during waiting list conditions. All these findings bear out the logic of the 'coping cycle' analysis and substantiate the predictions made by Billings and Moos (1981) in discussing their CRQ measure. Furthermore, improved coping skills may imply less problems in the future. This may turn out to be the main consequence of seeing a psychologist, as opposed to simply accelerating an existing process of improvement.

As Billings and Moos (1981) have pointed out, personal coping skills may only be part of the explanation for the client's improvement. It is plausible that informal 'social support' was also activated by formal therapy sessions (Holahan and Moos, 1981). In the original CRQ study Billings and Moos (1981) found that social support and coping skills played equal and overlapping parts in moderating stress. This possibility will be investigated in a subsequent study closely linked to the present one.

The relatively small mean changes in the CRQ scores also raises questions about the advisability of measuring coping with this instrument. One possible reason for the small change, identified by Billings and Moos (1981, p. 145), is that 'the use of one coping response may be sufficient to reduce stress and thus lessen the need to use other responses'. In this sense, large changes in individual questionnaire items may easily be obscured by small changes in the remaining items, when mean results are considered.

A related problem is that the CRQ was standardised on a non-clinical sample. As a consequence there are no items referring to the kind of coping skills that were introduced in therapy for a clinical sample, such as progressive muscular relaxation or response prevention.

It is important that we grapple with these problems, for a number of reasons. One reason is that changes in personal coping strategies seem to result in far more substantial improvements than those procured by medication and the other variables operating during waiting list conditions. One implication of this impact is that practitioners who work in this way do far more than simply act as catalysts, accelerating an existing recovery process. This interpretation dramatically affects economic calculations (e.g. Robson et al., 1984) because of the much greater relative benefit obtained through this kind of intervention.

Another reason for studying coping skills is the implication that follows for the maintenance and generalisation of clinical improvements: even if this kind of therapy only catalysed in the short term, it might still be justified on the basis of longer-term effects. To return to social support, it may be that our clients share their newly acquired and refined coping skills with relatives and friends. In turn this may influence how they use mental health services. To illustrate, we had recurring anecdotal evidence from our clients that they had indeed shared some of their coping skills with family and friends. Moreover, they often judged that their 'informal psychotherapy' had been successful. In short, we need to study our interventions in much greater detail than heretofore. As Willems (1973) has illustrated from the many unexpected lessons of ecology, short-term good may often be overturned by long-term harm. It seems that the study of personal coping skills provides an opportunity for us to learn about our therapeutic interventions so that we can perhaps minimise some of the man-made disasters Willems discussed, and maximise our service to the client.

One next step along these lines is to expand the CRQ so that it incorporates items obviously represented in therapy, utilise the measure in a longitudinal study like this one, then to conduct a discriminant analysis so as to determine which items are actually important in samples of clients who improve and those who do not. This may tell us quite a lot about the relation between client characteristics, the actual effect of therapy on coping and the kinds of coping skills that are valuable with given clinical problems. In turn, this could provide a very valuable guide to therapists and a more efficient service to clients.

Finally, we turn to the 'consumer satisfaction' results (SEQ). These findings suggested that the service was very acceptable to clients. The aims and methods which were used were particularly highly endorsed. Slightly less satisfaction was expressed regarding the content and outcome aspects. Those findings urge us to study in greater detail what it is that is seen as unacceptable by clients. 'Feedback' from this source may well complement the guidance we can obtain from a better measurement of coping.

Nonetheless, the general level of client satisfaction is high, and bears comparison with the results from other services. Paykel and Griffith (1983), for instance, used a similar seven-point rating scale with over 50 patients seeing CPNs or psychiatrists. They reported mean general satisfaction ratings of 1.8 and 2.8, respectively. However, the 13 items in their 'consumer satisfaction schedule' were confined to therapist qualities, or what we have referred to as 'process' variables in our SEQ measure. It is not possible, therefore, to compare client ratings on the other variables. The same problem prevents comparisons being made with the previous evaluations made by psychologists and their work, although in general the high level of satisfaction discussed above appears very similar to that reported by other psychologists (e.g. Earll and Kincey, 1982; Freeman and Button, 1984).

In conclusion, this evaluation fulfilled much of the promise outlined in Chapters 1 and 2. It helped us to develop our under-standing of the service we provided, and its respective effects on the clients' 'stress' and 'strain'. This in turn allowed us to evaluate whether the service was achieving its original goal of a significant clinical improvement brought about by increasing coping skills. The evidence suggested that it did indeed do so, in the predicted fashion. The implication was that our 'coping cycle' analysis was valid and worth pursuing. One obvious avenue to explore is in refining the coping instrument so as to include more of the skills relevant to the given therapy. In addition, it seems important to consider informal 'social support' alongside an individual's formally honed coping skills, so that we obtain a better grasp of their relationship and can adapt our service accordingly (Gottlieb, 1983).

This evaluation also suggests that the clients were different from those studied by Robson *et al.* (1984), in that they did not show any sign of getting better without specialist help. Thus, their relatively pessimistic assessment of the value of seeing a psychologist (namely that this accelerated but did not ultimately alter the outcome when clients were assessed after 1 year) may be valid only for the less chronic sample that they seem to have studied. However, the present evaluation only considered a 5-month 'control' period, in contrast to the 12 months covered by the Robson *et al.* (1984) assessment. Hence, it is premature to speculate further on this very substantial implication for the work of psychologists until more data are to hand. We hope to report such data in the near future, contrasting the present evaluation with one pursued in a GP surgery with a sample and time scale more akin to that of Robson *et al.* (1984).

ACKNOWLEDGEMENTS

This study entailed considerable assistance in organising, administering, scoring, analysing and summarising the measures. For their invaluable assistance in this work I am indebted to Eileen Greaves, Trish Harrison, Keith Henshall, Fiona Castle, Julie Sowery and Judy Milne. My former colleague Rosemary Jones collaborated in the project initially and provided helpful comments, as did Stephen Morley, Iain Burnside, Anne Broadhurst, Keith Turner, Carolyn Ainscough and Stuart Linke.

REFERENCES

Agras, W.S. and Berkowitz, R. (1980) 'Clinical Research in Behavior Therapy: Halfway There?', *Behavior Therapy, 11*, 472-87

Banks, M.H., Clegg, C.W., Jackson, P.R., Kemp, N.J., Stafford, E.M. and Wall, T.D. (1980) 'The Use of the General Health Questionnaire as an Indicator of Mental Health in Occupational Studies', *Journal of Occupational Psychology, 53*, 187-94

Barlow, D.H., Hayes, S.C. and Nelson, R.O. (1984) *The Scientist–Practitioner*, Pergamon, New York

Beck, A.T., Ward, C.H., Mendelson, M., Mock, J. and Erbaugh, J. (1961) 'An Inventory for Measuring Depression', *Archives of General Psychiatry, 4*, 53-63

Beck, A.T. (1979). *Cognitive Therapy of Depression*, Guilford Press, New York

Billings, A.G. and Moos, R.H. (1981) 'The Role of Coping Responses and Social Resources in Attenuating the Stress of Life Events', *Journal of Behavioural Medicine, 4*, 139-57

Brooker, C. and Wiggins, R.D. (1983). 'Nurse Therapist Trainee Variability: the Implications of Selection and Training', *Journal of Advanced Nursing, 8*, 321-8

Clark, D.F. (1979) 'The Clinical Psychologist in Primary Care', *Social Science of Medicine, 13A*, 707-13

Cohen, F. and Lazarus, R.S. (1979). 'Coping with Stresses of Illness', in: G.C. Stone, F.Cohen and N.E. Adler (eds), *Health Psychology: A Handbook*, Jossey Bass, London

Cohen, L.H. (1976) 'Clinicians' Utilization of Research Findings', *JSAS Catalog of Selected Documents in Psychology, 6*, 116

Cowen, E.L., Lorion, R.P. and Dorr, D. (1974) 'Research in the

Community Cauldron: a Case History', *Canadian Psychologist*, *15*, 313-25

Davidson, A.F. (1977) 'Clinical Psychology and General Practice: A Preliminary Inquiry', *Bulletin of the British Psychological Society*, *30*, 337-8

Durham, R.C. and Turvey, A.A. (1986) 'Cognitive Versus Behaviour Therapy in the Treatment of Chronic General Anxiety: Outcome at Discharge and at Six Month Follow-up. Paper presented at the Annual Conference of the BABP, Manchester

Earll, L. and Kincey, J. (1982) 'Clinical Psychology in General Practice: A Controlled Trial Evaluation', *Journal of the Royal College of General Practitioners*, *32*, 32-7

Firth, J. and Shapiro, D.A. (1986) 'An Evaluation of Psychotherapy for Job-related Distress', *Journal of Occupational Psychology*, *59*, 111-19

Freeman, G.K. and Button, E.J. (1984) 'The Clinical Psychologist in General Practice: A Six Year Study of Consulting Patterns for Psychosocial Problems' *Journal of the Royal College of General Practitioners*, *34*, 377-80

Gottlieb, B.H. (1983) *Social Support Strategies: Guidelines for Mental Health Practice*, Sage, London

Hawks, D. (1981) 'The Dilemma of Clinical Practice: Surviving as a Clinical Psychologist', in: I. McPherson and A. Sutton (eds), *Reconstructing Psychological Practice*, Croom Helm, London

Hodgson, R.J. and Rachman, S. (1977) 'Obsessional–Compulsive Complaints', *Behaviour Research and Therapy*, *15*, 389-95

Holahan, C.J. and Moos, R.H. (1981) 'Social Support and Psychological Distress: A Longitudinal Analysis', *Journal of Abnormal Psychology*, *90*, 365-70

Ives, G. (1979) 'Psychological Treatment in General Practice', *Journal of the Royal College of General Practitioners*, *29*, 343-51

Jerrom, D.W.A., Simpson, R.J., Barber, J.H. and Pemberton, D.A. (1983) 'General Practitioners' Satisfaction with a Primary Care Clinical Psychology Service', *Journal of the Royal College of General Practitioners*, *33*, 29-31

Kanfer, F.H. and Saslow, G. (1969) 'Behavioral Diagnosis', in: C.M. Franks (ed.), *Behavior Therapy: Appraisal and Status*, McGraw-Hill, New York

Koch, H.C.H. (1979) 'Evaluation of Behaviour Therapy Intervention in General Practice', *Journal of the Royal College of General Practitioners*, *29*, 337-40

Marks, I.M. (1985) *Psychiatric Nurse Therapists in Primary Care*, Royal College of Nursing, London

Marks, I.M. and Mathews, A.M. (1979) 'Brief Standard Self-rating for Phobic Patients', *Behaviour Research and Therapy*, *17*, 263-7

Milne, D.L. (1986) *Training Behaviour Therapists: Methods, Evaluation and Implementation with Parents, Nurses and Teachers*, Croom Helm, London/Brookline Books, Cambridge, Mass.

Milne, D.L. and Castle, F. (1986) 'A Process Evaluation of a Routine Out-Patient Service'. Paper presented at the Annual Conference of the

British Association for Behavioural Psychotherapy, Manchester

Milne, D.L. and Linford, J. (1984) *Anxiety: How to Understand and Control your Nerves.* MIND (National Association for Mental Health), Wakefield Branch

Moos, R.H. (ed.) (1976) *Human Adaption: Coping with Life Crises.* D.C. Heath, Lexington, Mass.

McPherson, I.G. and Feldman, M.P. (1977) 'A Preliminary Investigation of the Role of the Clinical Psychologist in the Primary Care Setting', *Bulletin of the British Psychological Society, 30,* 342-6

Paykel, E.S. and Griffith, J.H. (1983) *Community Psychiatric Nursing for Neurotic Patients,* Royal College of Nursing, London

Pearlin, L.I. and Schooler, C. (1983) 'The Structure of Coping', *Journal of Health and Social Behaviour, 19,* 2-21

Peterson, L., Homer, A.L. and Wonderlich, S.A. (1982) 'The Integrity of Independent Variables in Behavior Analysis', *Journal of Applied Behavior Analysis, 15,* 477-92

Redfield, J.R. and Stone, A. (1979) 'Individual Viewpoints of Stressful Life Events', *Journal of Consulting and Clinical Psychology, 47,* 147-54

Robson, M.H., France, R. and Bland, M. (1984) 'Clinical Psychologist in Primary Care: Controlled Clinical and Economic Evaluation', *British Medical Journal, 288,* 1805-8

Shepherd, M., Cooper, B., Brown, A.C. and Kalton, G. (1966) *Psychiatric Illness in General Practice,* Oxford University Press, London

Tennant, C. and Andrews, G. (1976) 'A Scale to Measure the Stress of Life Events', *Australian and New Zealand Journal of Psychiatry, 10,* 27-32

Watts, F.N. (1985) 'Clinical Psychology', *Health Trends, 17,* 28-31

Willems, E.P. (1973) 'Go Ye into all the World and Modify Behaviour: An Ecologist's View', *Representative Research in Social Psychology, 4,* 93-105

Wolf, M.M. (1978) 'Social Validity: The Case for a Subjective Measurement or how Applied Behavior Analysis is finding its Heart', *Journal of Applied Behavior Analysis, 11,* 203-14

7

Evaluation in Community Psychiatric Nursing

David Skidmore

EDITOR'S INTRODUCTION

David Skidmore's chapter draws attention to an all too common phenomenon, the detachment of service planning from objective data. While this practice has greatly increased the number of community psychiatric nurses (CPNs) in post in the short term, Skidmore suggests that this has been based on a wishful assumption that CPNs are some kind of psychiatric panacea. He argues that future developments of CPN services should be based on a marriage of everyday practice and evaluative research.

The particularly crucial research topics he identifies are to examine the variety of presenting problems, to conduct an analysis of the skills practitioners need to assist with these problems, and to determine the resources required to support the application of these skills. Case studies of each topic are provided.

Skidmore suggests that an emphasis on marrying practice and research in this way will help CPNs to play a central role in the great advances that can be made in the long term.

In 1966, in the UK 46 psychiatric hospitals offered a community psychiatric nursing (CPN) service. By 1980 this had risen to 163 services. Similarly, by 1985 there were some 3000 CPNs in the UK, most services having doubled their numbers over the last 10 years. In some areas an additional increase of up to 300 per cent is forecast by 1990.

Despite this 'coming of age', very little research has been carried out concerning the effectiveness of a CPN service. This is not to say that the arena of community psychiatric nursing is under-researched; indeed one can discover a myriad of titles in the literature. Unfortunately the majority of these articles tend to be subjective in nature and, whilst useful in contributing to the overall picture of the CPN, they offer little information regarding the evaluation of the service. A glance through this literature illustrates the implicit rationale that it is generally accepted that community psychiatric nursing is the answer to all psychiatric problems. There are, however, too few evaluative studies that support such notions; too few comparisons between community and traditional psychiatric care; too little effort given over to the identification of client needs. Despite this dearth of data the assumption that the CPN is the 'ideal' caregiver is adding weight to the argument for 'de-institutionalisation'. Consequently, rather than being a review of previous studies, this section is more a cry for action. Hopefully it will identify some of the areas worthy of examination by the practitioners, and offer guidelines so that these areas can be effectively researched.

7.1 PROMINENT EVALUATION THEMES

The main focus of attention apparent from the few research projects tends to be concerned with the nature of the service, rather than the outcome from that service. Consequently one can quite easily identify differences between individual services from the literature, without gaining any insight into the consequences of intervention. The question of CPN location is a major concern (Leopoldt, 1975; Shaw, 1977; Sharpe, 1982) and interest in this area has initiated the argument for location within the primary health care team (PHCT). Whilst one accepts that there is a need for such a location (Skidmore, 1980), little evidence has been offered to support the CPN's effectiveness in such an arena. We do not know the type of skills that he/she would need, nor do we know the kinds of resources that such a base would demand. It has been argued that such a location would do no more than extend the institution into the community (Golan, 1978). To counter such suggestions evidence to the contrary is certainly required.

Evaluation of the CPN's role is a theme which has claimed interest only in recent years, and is offering a steady trickle of

145

information concerning the need for skills training and effective supervision. Many of these studies are not yet published but are eagerly awaited.

However, the important areas of client satisfaction and client needs have attracted very little interest, and it is in this field where the most useful advances can be made and are needed. One study that did consider client satisfaction was that carried out by Milne, Walker and Bentinck (1985). This suggested that a partnership in therapy, between client and therapist, was a viable alternative to the traditional 'mechanistic' form of intervention. Their findings endorsed the conclusion of Skidmore and Stoker (1974), that the involvement of the client in therapeutic decision-making and the use of self-assessment can potentiate the effects of intervention strategies.

Paykel and Griffith (1983) also examined the level of client satisfaction. Their study, although confined to one particular area (Wandsworth and Merton in south-west London) and concentrating on a specific clientele (neurotics), is an excellent example of evaluative techniques. Their study compared the CPN service with that of 'traditional' outpatient care and used a modified control trial design. An abridged version of their study would not do justice to the findings, and readers are urged to read the full report. Paykel and Griffith suggested that CPNs produced greater client satisfaction than traditional outpatient care, although no significant differences were identified in the efficacy of both services. However, CPNs appeared to produce a reduction in client contact with other agencies; achieved greater discharge rates; and provided a more economic service in the long term. They concluded that the CPN offered a valuable mode of care.

It could be suggested that Paykel and Griffith is an essential 'read' for the prospective evaluative researcher, since they offer a helpful breakdown of the method and research tools used. Certainly, replication of this study in other areas would be of great value to the overall pool of knowledge regarding community psychiatric nursing.

Similarly Butterworth (1986) has approached community psychiatric nursing from a position favourable to the client. He examined the outcome of intervention by offering a 'problem-centred' approach. He suggested that the CPN experiences difficulty when asked to describe case-work and that this difficulty could be overcome with a better theoretical stance.

Skidmore and Friend (1984) would endorse these findings following their study of twelve CPN teams. They concluded that CPNs lack the necessary training that their roles demand, and suggest a radical change in their education.

7.2 METHODS OF CHOICE

The studies outlined above have reflected many of the research methods on offer. Non-participative observations appear to be the most common methods used when attempting to gather information on what CPNs actually do. Obviously such methods are fraught with problems, particularly that problem which allows one to see only that which one chooses to see (Lippman, 1922). Milne *et al.* (1985) and Butterworth (1986) used more complex but more reliable methods, ones which enter the realms of 'action' research. Both studies relied on continuous assessment of subjects and outcome, and involved quite useful record-keeping. The Milne study is particularly interesting in that it utilised therapist ratings and client self-rating for comparison. This method is valuable not only in identifying progress, but also in maintaining client participation in therapy.

Skidmore and Friend (1984) used a combination of methods to examine several issues over a 3-year period: content analysis of referral records, to identify reasons for referral and new cases; observations so that intervention techniques could be identified; and open interviews in an attempt to identify the CPNs' needs. The major difficulty with this study was that one could not control for the 'best performance pantomime', when subjects know that they are being observed.

7.3 SUGGESTED DIRECTIONS

Previous literature suggests that there are several directions that evaluative research can take in the field of community psychiatric nursing, all of equal importance. The process of de-institutionalisation is with us, along with a significant increase in the numbers of practising CPNs. In order to develop an effective service to their clients, CPNs need to examine certain crucial issues:

(1) the varieties of presenting problems demanding intervention;
(2) the skills needed to meet that demand;
(3) the type of resources required to deliver such skills effectively.

In an attempt to identify these areas, and how they might be approached, I intend to describe three illustrative studies. Each study was evaluative in nature and considered the client's position from quite different standpoints.

1. Doyle (1982) suggested that the CPN could instigate improvement in those clients dependent upon 'minor' psychotropic drugs, if based within the PHCT. His rationale had its genesis in the analysis of the prescribing habits of the general practitioner and led to the suggestion that many of the drugs prescribed were unnecessary. He argued that the location of a CPN within the PHCT, functioning in an advisory/counselling position, would negate much of the need for these drugs. In order to test this theory he intended to compare two 'matched-subject' groups. This design requires the researcher to allocate clients evenly to both of the studied groups in terms of important variables, such as diagnosis or chronicity. In Doyle's study one group had access to the counsellor–CPN while the other had traditional GP care. A record of presenting symptoms, prescriptions and psychiatric referral rates were to be maintained for future comparison. The outcome of such a study could prove invaluable to the development of community psychiatric nursing, offering vital information concerning the role and educational requirements of the CPN. Should the CPN prove to be effective in this area it would help to reduce the demands upon GPs' time and create economical saving via the reduction in drug usage. The role that the CPN can play in the PHCT is one area worthy of further investigation.

On the other hand, Freeman and Button (1984) suggested that there is a natural decline in the prescription rates for patients with psychosocial problems in general practice. They argue that such problems do not benefit from individual therapy because of a natural pattern of crisis and remission. This study may appear to contradict Doyle's preliminary findings but neither study is directly comparable. Doyle was specifically focusing on the *pattern* of prescription, whereas Freeman and Button were more interested in the prescriptions that occurred during therapeutic encounters. They mentioned that they referred to the practice records for other information in this area, but do not mention whether or not they took into account the 'maintenance prescriptions' offered in some practices (often for 6-month medication courses). Again, despite their suggestion of a natural decline, the figures in their study suggest that prescription rates plateau rather than reduce. More important they imply that the prescription rate reduced more in the study group than it did in the total practice population. Consequently we are presented with a problem of methodology, since there is no 'control' group with whom to compare the overall results of therapy. To avoid such difficulties it is essential to collect comparable records with an 'untreated' population so that the full impact of intervention can be evaluated.

2. *Friend (1984)* provided an illustration of the second issue identified earlier, that of the skills required to develop an effective CPN service. He was more concerned with attempting to prevent readmission rates within the existing psychiatric population; whereas Doyle focused on the 'acute' area, Friend was concerned with what he terms 'chronic psychological dysfunction'. His preliminary observations suggested that re-admissions had little to do with a client's psychological condition, and were the result of the family's inability to cope with a 'spoiled identity' within their midst. Adopting a 'matched-subject' design like Doyle's, Friend felt that the role of the CPN in terms of mental health education could be evaluated. One group of CPNs would function as 'educators' and use family members as co-therapists, whereas the other group would continue in their usual manner. This comparison was based on his initial findings which implied that CPNs, in the area he was studying, rarely involved the family in discussion or therapy. Comparison of re-admission rates and the satisfaction of both family and client (in terms of outcome) were then to be compared. Again, such a study could hold important implications concerning the future role of the CPN.

3. Turning to our third identified issue, *Smith (1980)* planned to evaluate the psychiatric needs of those within inner-city areas by eliciting the client's definitions of needs. Topics included care and resources, and the identification of how far these needs could be accommodated within the traditional and

the community models of care. He also intended to compare clients' accounts of outcome satisfaction from both arenas.

7.4 DISCUSSION

The studies outlined above could provide the information required to build the foundations of an effective service. Rather than progressing in an *ad hoc* manner, as seems to be the case today, CPNs need the information that can systematically direct their professional development. I would argue that credible information can only be collected by a programme of evaluative research, as indicated by the studies outlined above.

The prime concern of CPNs should be the quality of care that they can offer to the client. The development of that quality cannot be made without evaluating the needs of the client, and those needs cannot be identified or evaluated by observation alone. Milne *et al.* (1985) propose an excellent method of evaluation which marries intervention, research and client participation together. The type of approach that this study used could be adopted, so that practice and data collection walk hand in hand. What is particularly impressive about this approach is that it can maintain objectivity in both practice and data recording, since the ultimate interpretation of each is not the responsibility of one single person. The results could also offer some direction on the future training needs of CPNs, and the type of resources required for effective practice.

Much more information is needed of similar quality if CPNs are to develop professionally. One could suggest that since the CPN is in the front line of the de-institutionalisation programme they must 'arm' effectively. Knowledge of the outcome of actions is necessary to do this, as is knowledge of the potential clientele. There are several effective ways of gaining this information; that indicated by Milne *et al.* (1985) and Butterworth (1986), as well as those methods developed from practice. The accurate recording of case histories/studies is an effective way of evaluating interventions, when coupled with client participation. Such a method would provide a means of on-going evaluation of intervention strategy and client satisfaction.

Another area worthy of research concerns the feasibility of community care. If one considers the experiences of America and Italy regarding de-institutionalisation, then it is imperative that those benefiting most from community care should have the opportunity to receive it. Conversely, those who would be disadvantaged by being placed back in the community should have the choice of environment that most suits them, even if this means retaining hospital beds. This is one of the issues that has received minimal attention. In many respects the development of community psychiatric care has been the produce of armchair speculation. The professionals decide what is best for their clients and act accordingly, in much the same way that hospitalisation was enforced on the psychiatric population. Any action that directly affects a client should be taken through partnership, and that means respecting the needs and wishes of clients. It has been illustrated that commitment to decisions is greatly enhanced when all parties concerned take part in that decision (Gellerman, 1974).

It could be argued that the environment in which 'therapy' takes place is an extension of the therapy and can, accordingly, enhance or hamper progress. The feelings that clients have towards their treatment environments has been illustrated by Skidmore (1980) in a study that compared anxiety levels of clients entering medical encounters in the community and those having encounters in the hospital. Certain key points can be noted from this study:

(1) The treatment/consulting environment was important. Some buildings are symbolic in that they convey 'intention'. Consider the example of being 'sent', by your GP, to see a specialist at the hospital. The implication of this action is that one is ill, since one is being sent to a place that specialises in treating illness. Furthermore, the hospital may have a reputation for certain specialisms, and can suggest to the clients that they too have a certain disease.
(2) Negative expectations develop during encounters in which little information is offered. Such expectations can impair progress of any treatment (Bradshaw, 1978).
(3) Using various research methods to gather data about one area can lead to a more accurate evaluation.

In short, when approaching community psychiatric nursing from a research point of view, the influence of all parties concerned must be considered. Similarly, all those factors that influence the individual (experience, biographies, age) must also be considered.

If the complications that occurred during the institutionalisation process are to be avoided in the community then information regarding the implications of community care and its alternatives are required. The CPN should utilise the expertise of other professionals in order to collect this information.

7.5 CONCLUSION

Community psychiatric nursing is progressing at a rapid pace with very serious implications for standards of care, education and resources. Those involved with, and committed to, the service should not allow it to progress in an *ad hoc* manner, at the whim of armchair speculators, but should involve themselves with that development. By marrying a process of evaluative research with everyday practice, great advances can be made. Some of the areas much in need of investigation have been identified above, along with some methodological guidelines. The practitioner is in the best position to carry out future studies and could participate in his/her own development much more effectively.

REFERENCES

Bradshaw, J. (1978) *Doctors on Trial*, Wildwood Press, London
Butterworth, C.A. (1986) 'New Technologies within Organisations in Transition', unpublished Ph.D. thesis, Aston University, Birmingham
Doyle, C. (1982) 'A Scheme to Reduce Psychotrophic Drug Prescription', unpublished M.Phil. thesis, Manchester Polytechnic
Friend, W. (1984) 'Re-admission: Psychological or Sociological Dysfunction', unpublished M.Phil. thesis, Manchester Polytechnic
Freeman, G.K. and Button, E.J. (1984) 'The Clinical Psychologist in General Practice', *Journal of the Royal College of General Practitioners, 34*, pp. 377-80
Golan, N. (1978) *Treatment in Crisis Situations*, Macmillan, London
Gellerman, S. (1974) *The Behavioural Science in Management*, Penguin, Harmondsworth, UK
Leopoldt, H. (1975) 'Attachment and Psychiatric Domiciliary Attachment', *Nursing Mirror, 141*, pp. 82-4

Lippman, W. (1922) *Public Opinion*, Macmillan, London

Milne, D., Walker, J. and Bentinck, V. (1985) 'The Value of Feedback', *Nursing Times, 81*, pp. 34-6

Paykel, E.S. and Griffith, J.H. (1983) *Community Psychiatric Nursing for Neurotic Patients*, Royal College of Nursing, London

Sharpe, D. (1982) 'GP's views of Community Psychiatric Nurses', *Nursing Times, 78*, pp. 1664-6

Shaw, A. (1977) 'CPN Attachment in Group Practice', *Nursing Times* (Health Care Supplement), *73*, p. 12

Skidmore, D. (1980) *The Hidden Machine*, Verus Microfiche, Bournemouth

Skidmore, D. and Friend, W. (1984) 'Muddling Through', *Community Outlook*, 9 May, pp. 179-81

Skidmore, D. and Stoker, M.J. (1974) 'Space Age Therapy', *New Psychiatry, 1*, pp. 179-81

Smith, C. (1980) 'Traditional or Community Care: The Inner City Needs', unpublished M.Phil. thesis, Manchester Polytechnic

8

Evaluation in Drama Therapy

Roger Grainger

EDITOR'S INTRODUCTION

Like the preceding chapter, the present one shares a concern
for the disproportionate attention accorded in the literature
to describing the kind of work practitioners undertake, at the
expense of evaluating this effort. Roger Grainger provides an
illustration of how the balance can be restored. He describes
a careful analysis of the relative effects of routine day hospital attendance versus day hospital plus drama therapy. The
outcome measure was the thought disorder test, and the
subjects were twelve successive day hospital referrals. The
results suggested that in both groups the construct systems of
individual patients improved, underlining the need for
systematic evaluation to tease out the incremental effects of
novel therapies.

Accounts of the therapeutic effects of drama therapy tend to be
somewhat vague, often couched in psychoanalytic language
about the achievement of catharsis and the integration of
repressed material within consciousness — effects which are
difficult to quantify (although not impossible, with the help of
projective techniques). The use of drama in order to increase
people's ability to give cognitive structure to their perception of
other people suggests the use of techniques which produce
results which may be more readily evaluated.

8.1 DRAMA AND INVOLVEMENT

Drama therapy is the use of dramatic experience to heal people.

154

This does not mean that the things that happen in a drama therapy programme are in the ordinary sense 'dramatic'. Indeed, they can sometimes appear to be rather dull! It refers instead to the mechanisms underlying actual dramatic presentation. In other words, drama therapy concentrates upon the universal human experience of sharing or involvement which allows people to 'put themselves in the place of' the characters in a play and so gain a temporary release from the pressure of their own preoccupations. In a strange way the play allows those involved to 'be themselves' — that is, to express feelings and attitudes which are habitually unacknowledged — while they are pretending to be 'someone else'. This may be because of a particular way of experiencing reality characteristic of drama in which our awareness *oscillates*, so that we alternately stand back from and immerse ourselves in what is taking place in front of or around us (Buber, 1957; May, 1975). The feelings of satisfaction and serenity which come from a play that 'moves' us have to do with losing our separate individual identities in a shared experience of life, while our ability to integrate these feelings and to translate them into ideas that we can use for the future belongs to the movement of withdrawal and detachment in which we understand that 'it's only a play', and perhaps begin to experience 'real life' a little differently. Both movements are necessary; without the possibility of withdrawing we would never allow ourselves to get involved and run the risk of forfeiting our independent selfhood. Within the structure of the play we feel both safe and challenged. Drama makes a firm distinction between two kinds of reality, and tells us clearly that neither of them has a final hold over us (Wilshire, 1982). Within the limits of a structure which is clearly perceived and understood, it provides a comparatively safe 'middle ground' between private fantasy and public reality (Winnicott, 1971), allowing a limited 'engulfment' in other people, and a ready-made identity within an obvious structure (Moreno, 1972; Jennings, 1985; Schattner and Courtney, 1981).

8.2 DRAMA THERAPY AND SCHIZOPHRENIA

Whether schizophrenic thinking is characterised as excessively narrow, limited and concrete, or as too broad, generalised and over-inclusive, there is general agreement that thought-disordered people have difficulties in distinguishing those boundaries of self and other which structure human relationships. There is difficulty in discriminating between subject and object, self-as-participant and self-as-observer, and in categorising different degrees of involvement and concern. In such cases, says Johnson, 'the therapeutic goal is to reverse the vicious circle of primary boundary confusion anxiety and retreat from reality' by providing an environment with 'distinct boundaries and structure to ensure that the insecure personality will not be engulfed' (1981, p. 30). In the next section we shall be looking at an investigation which aimed to provide this kind of setting in drama therapy terms, and to examine the effect of drama therapy on the way we structure our perception of the world.

8.3 AN INVESTIGATION INTO THE EFFECT OF DRAMA THERAPY ON CONSTRUCT FORMATION

(a) Introduction

Almost all the studies of drama therapy are content to expound the underlying theory and describe what takes place during sessions without venturing into the more hazardous area of evaluating results (see Mazer, 1982; Johnson, 1982; Landy, 1982; Emunah, 1983; Rayner, 1984; see also Schattner and Courtney, 1981; and Langley, 1983). An exception is an assessment of drama therapy in a child guidance setting carried out in 1972 by Irwin, Levy and Shapiro, which used a projective test, the Rorschach Index of Repressive Style, and measures of linguistic ability to evaluate the effect of a programme of drama therapy (an RTRS score indicates the extent to which images, emotions and past experiences are verbally labelled and thus available in consciousness in communicable terms). The results indicated that 'drama therapy was an effective therapeutic technique', significantly lessening repression and increasing verbal fluency. On the other hand, when Spencer, Gillespie and Ekisa (1983) used members of a drama therapy programme as a control group for an investigation into the effectiveness of social skills training according to a behaviour modification model, only the social skills training resulted in significant improvement. Subjects in this case were chronic schizophrenics, all of whom had been patients in a psychiatric hospital for several years. The aim of the treatment programme was to improve their 'conversation skills', which the social-skills training did quite effectively.

Believing that drama therapy has more to do with organising thoughts than extending people's conversational repertoire, a colleague, Mary Duggan, and myself carried out an investigation in a psychiatric day hospital which made use of personal construct theory to provide a way of evaluating drama therapy. The work of Bannister (1960, 1962, 1963, 1965; Bannister and Fransella 1966; Bannister, Adams-Webber, Pen and Radley 1975) suggests the suitability of personal construct theory for the interpretation and evaluation of psychodrama itself.

(b) Method

Subjects

The programme was included in the therapeutic services provided by a day hospital, care being taken not to present it as any kind of 'experiment'. There was no attempt to select people diagnosed as thought-disordered. Twelve subjects were included (nine female and three male), ranging in age between 38 and 75, each of whom had attained a score of over 8 on the vocabulary subscale of the Wechsler Adult Intelligence Scale. Selection was by successive referral — new patients arriving at the hospital were assigned to one of two treatment groups on a 'first-come, first-served' basis. (This reflects the policy of the day hospital, and also accords well with drama therapy, which requires a good 'mix' of personalities and an unclinical atmosphere of spontaneity.)

Procedure

Both groups received a course of drama therapy consisting of ten 1-hour sessions taking place twice a week, arranged in ascending degree of difficulty for thought-disordered people.

The exercises were intended to provide experience in being involved, and involving others, in imagined situations specially contrived to draw attention to the relationship between different kinds of personal reality, thus producing what Cox (1978) has called 'a complex differential empathy'. An example of a drama therapy session, taken from halfway through the course (Session 6) is briefly described:

(1) Whole group: Say hello to people in some way that will make them feel better. What did we do last week? How do you feel about it now?

(2) Partners: Put your partner in a pose characteristic of him/ her. Walk around and inspect the 'statues'. Wind them up and set them moving. Put your partner in an uncharacteristic pose; inspect, animate. Reverse whole process, swapping roles.

(3) Two groups: Each group chooses an emotion and forms itself into a group sculpture expressing it. Next, a group transforms itself into a sculpture expressing the opposite emotion. The other group guesses the emotions thus 'sculpted'. (This is to be done twice.)

(4) Whole group: Each member writes down the name of a feeling; the papers are shuffled, and each person draws one. What kind of thing makes you feel like this? The second time round, each speaks 'as if' he/she were his/her neighbour.

(5) Whole group: Everyone says goodbye to everyone else.

Design

A 'cross-over' design was adopted for the experiment. During the first 5 weeks Group 'A' received treatment but not Group 'B'; during the second 5 weeks Group 'B' but not Group 'A'. All subjects were tested three times; to begin with, and before and after the second group's sessions. (In this way everybody involved received the benefit of the treatment, and delayed or transitory effects could be noted.) A change in the direction of increased intensity and consistency of construing was predicted, as measured by the thought disorder test (Bannister and Fransella, 1966).

(c) Results

As was to be expected, the baseline testing showed subjects occupying different positions on the 'looseness–tightness' of construing continuum. The results of the second administration of the thought-disorder test showed a treatment effect for Group 'A' which was significant at the 5 per cent level (t-test, repeated measures) in the case of the intensity score. This was maintained at a slightly lower level 5 weeks later. Group 'B', however, also showed an increase (non-significant) in construct intensity during its period as a control group — which seems to reflect well upon the day hospital as a therapeutic environment. There were no significant differences in the scores for consistency. It is perhaps also of clinical relevance that three subjects who registered scores at the first testing which were low enough to suggest the presence of actual thought disorder had lifted well clear of the thought disorder criterion score by the second testing. The scores are summarised in Table 8.1.

Table 8.1:

	Mean intensity scores				Mean consistency scores		
Testing							
	1	2	3		1	2	3
	A	B	A		B		
A	11.52	16.71*	16.55	A	0.78	0.75	0.76
B	13.79	16.02	16.48	B	0.81	0.76	0.71
	5 weeks	5 weeks			5 weeks	5 weeks	

Between the first and second testing, A was the experimental group; between the second and third testing, B was the experimental group.
*Significant at 5 per cent level.

(d) Discussion

As predicted, significant improvements were obtained in the patients' construing of other people following drama therapy. However, the marked trend in the control (or 'B') group towards improved performance indicates that day hospital attendance contributed to this finding. It would seem that drama therapy may therefore enhance existing benefits of attendance, although a truly untreated control group would be required to give this interpretation more substance.

The results from Group 'B' reveal the sudden invalidation of part of an individual's construct system within the course of a single testing, which is associated with clinical depression (Bannister, 1960). Although this only occurred in one out of a group of six subjects, the statistical effect is dramatic. This illustrates the difficulties involved in trying to be experimentally rigorous in a setting in which rigid control of subjects can be counterproductive, particularly when dealing with a treatment modality which puts a high premium on spontaneity and freedom of expression (Grainger, 1985). Each of the participants was informed that he or she could decline to participate at any stage of the programme, and there was no attempt to subject them to any kind of selection process. The necessity of administering the thought disorder test tended to give an unwelcome 'clinical' flavour to the proceedings, and consequently some of the exercises were designed to produce results which could be compared and assimilated as part of the drama therapy sessions. For example an informal repertory grid was built into the exercise comprising the first and last sessions of each programme. Group 'A' refused to allow themselves to be scored, but Group 'B' produced a mean group intensity score of 178 at the last session, compared with 162 at the first one.

Certainly the investigation would benefit from using more subjects, but interesting clinical effects reveal themselves even when the statistical significance is not apparent, and it would be a pity to risk 'throwing the baby out with the bathwater' by trying to be too rigorous in applying scientific controls, and so inhibiting the behaviour to be studied. In this case the use of the thought disorder test seems particularly appropriate because it deals explicitly with the way people present themselves to, and are construed by, others and the test task (of sorting photographs and judging facial expressions) leads more or less naturally into exercises in personal interaction and relationship. Finally, the experiment may be said to have contributed to a very real improvement in patients' health brought about by the overall day hospital programme.

REFERENCES

Bannister, D. (1960) 'Conceptual Structure in Thought-disorder Schizophrenics', *Journal of Mental Science*, 106, pp. 1230-49

Bannister, D. (1962) 'The Nature and Measurement of Schizophrenic Thought-disorder', *Journal of Mental Science*, 106, pp. 824-42

Bannister, D. (1963) 'The Genesis of Schizophrenic Thought-disorder; A Serial Invalidation Hypothesis', *British Journal of Psychiatry*, 109, pp. 680-6

Bannister, D. (1965) 'The Genesis of Schizophrenic Thought-disorder; Re-test of the Serial Invalidation Hypothesis', *British Journal of Psychiatry*, 111, pp. 327-82

Bannister, D. and Fransella, F. (1966) 'A Grid Test of Schizophrenic Thought-disorder', *British Journal of Social and Clinical Psychology*, 5, pp. 95-102

Bannister, D., Adams-Webber, J.R., Pen, W.I. and Radley, A.R. (1975) 'Reversing the Process of Thought-disorder: A Serial Validation Experiment', *British Journal of Social and Clinical Psychology*, 14, pp. 169-80

Buber, M. (1957) *Pointing the Way*, Routledge & Kegan Paul, London

Cox, M. (1978) *Structuring the Therapeutic Process*, Pergamon, London and New York

Emunah, R. (1983) 'Drama Therapy with Adult Psychiatric Patients', *Arts in Psychiatry*, 10, pp. 77-89

Grainger, R. (1985) 'Using Drama Creatively in Therapy', *Drama Therapy*, 8, pp. 33-46

Irwin, C., Levy, P. and Shapiro, M. (1972) 'Assessment of Drama Therapy in a Child Guidance Setting', *Group Psychotherapy and Psychodrama*, 24, pp. 105-16

Jennings, S. (ed.) (1985) *Creative Therapy*, Kemble Press and Dramatherapy Consultants, St Albans, Herts.

Johnson, D.R. (1981) 'Developmental Approaches in Drama Therapy', *Arts in Psychiatry*, 9, pp. 183-9

Landy, R.J. (1982) 'Training the Drama Therapist — A Four-part Model', *Arts in Psychiatry*, 9, pp. 91-9

Langley, D. (1983) *Dramatherapy and Psychiatry*, Croom Helm, London

May, R. (1975) *The Courage to Create*, Collins, London

Mazer, R. (1982) 'Drama Therapy for the Elderly in a Day-centre', *Hospital and Community Psychiatry*, 33, pp. 577-9

Moreno, J.L. (1972) *Psychodrama*, 4th edn, Beacon House, New York

Rayner, P. (1984) 'Psychodrama as a Medium for Intermediate Treatment', *British Journal of Social Work*, 7, p. 4

Schattner, G. and Courtney, R. (eds) (1981) *Drama in Therapy*, vol. 2, Drama Book Specialists, New York

Spencer, P.G., Gillespie, C.R. and Ekisa, E.G.E. (1983) 'A Controlled Comparison of Social Skills Training and Remedial Drama on the Conversational Skills of Chronic Schizophrenic In-patients', *British Journal of Psychiatry*, 143, pp. 165-72

Wilshire, M. (1982) *Role Play and Identity*, Indiana University Press, Bloomington, Indiana

Winnicott, D.W. (1945) 'Primitive Emotional Development', in D.W. Winnicott (1958) *Collected Papers: Through Paediatrics to Psychology*, Tavistock, London and New York

Winnicott, D.W. (1971) *Playing and Reality*, Tavistock, London and New York

9

Evaluation in Nursing:
The Nurse as Behaviour Therapist

Philip Barker

EDITOR'S INTRODUCTION

The focus of this chapter is largely upon the training and evaluation of mental health personnel. As such, it is a clear illustration of the ways in which we can apply the principles of evaluative research to a variety of problems. There is a specified goal ('good clinical practice'), an enterprising training process and a system of objective monitoring which gives feedback to the training course.

However, Barker's chapter is also about the evolving role of the nurse behaviour therapist. In this regard it is an interesting account of the ever-changing demands and resources that affect mental health personnel. Such changes provide a relevant challenge to the utility of an evaluative approach.

Anyone who has heard Barker speak about nurse behaviour therapy will not be disappointed by this chapter. It reflects his usual punchy, stimulating perspective on key issues, allied to a wholesome dose of questioning, self-critical speculation. In his concluding remarks he anticipates that nurses will increasingly incorporate evaluation into their routine work, leading to further developments in what has already been a major and rapid role expansion.

9.1 INTRODUCTION

American clinical practice provides the earliest published report on the nurse working as a 'therapist' within a behavioural model of care (Ayllon and Michael, 1959). More than 10 years were to elapse before Marks described his experimental training programme with British nurses in the early 1970s (Marks, 1973). However, despite the American historical precedent, the concept of *behaviour therapy nursing* appears to have a stronger base within British mental health nursing. Why should this be the case? One answer may be found in the differences between British and American traditions of clinical practice. For instance Altschul has argued that psychiatric nursing in the United States was custodial and restrictive in nature, until fairly recently. Those few nurses who did develop therapeutic roles tended to concentrate upon individual psychotherapy, and were influenced strongly by the American tradition of dynamic psychotherapy. In contrast, Altschul sees British nurses as having been involved in 'psychotherapeutic' activity for much longer: 'controlling and influencing the behaviour of patients without mechanical restraint since at least the late 19th century' (Altschul, 1985, p. 5). It would appear, therefore, that American nurses might inhabit either of the following worlds: those specialised settings, many of them privately funded, where traditional psychotherapy is the dominant model; or the more custodial care systems associated with the state hospitals. British nurses, at least according to Altschul, have not been exposed to quite such a stark choice of clinical model. Instead, most nurses have trained and worked in environments where more pragmatic, eclectic approaches have held sway. Such practical 'empiricism' is widely accepted as the hallmark of the British psychiatric establishment: a feature which may have assisted the growth of behaviour therapy nursing which is also a largely pragmatic, eclectic model of care.

The primary aim of this chapter is to clarify our understanding of the term *behaviour therapy nursing*. Although the literature on evaluative research within this area of nursing is limited, I shall attempt to illustrate the major concerns of this facet of nursing practice, stressing both the goals and the methods of evaluation used. I shall also attempt to clarify the relationship between this field of research and mainstream clinical practice, ending with some suggestions about the further definition of the role of the 'nurse behaviour therapist'.

(a) The nurse as therapist

Perhaps the clearest description of the nurse as a 'behaviour therapist' in the early literature was made by Marks and his colleagues in a review of their training programme (Marks, Hallam, Connolly and Philpott, 1977). Their programme aimed to 'prepare nurses to work as *clinical specialists* in the administration of specific psychological treatments for *adult neurotics*, working as the main therapists in a psychiatric team and to carry more responsibility than usual' (my italics). It should be emphasised that the concept of behaviour therapy nursing under consideration in this chapter is broader in scope than that suggested by Marks *et al.* This concept would embrace nurses working as specialists, but would not exclude staff working within more traditional role models. Perhaps a more appropriate description of a nurse behaviour therapist would be: 'a nurse who has extended her/his role as a result of training in certain methods of assessment and behaviour change, and who works within a behavioural framework of care'. There is still some difficulty concerning the use of the term 'behavioural' since this has a wide range of meanings. Although the predominant theoretical orientation of the behaviour therapist's role is that of contemporary behaviourism, within recent years the behavioural approach has been influenced by, and subsequently accommodated, other models of care and treatment. (See Barker, 1982 for a discussion.) As a result, the practical work of the nurse behaviour therapist, as seen in this chapter, may be more flexible and broader in scope than that described by Marks and his colleagues. It will be argued that this model of nursing care is relevant not only to the care and treatment of adult neurotics, but to virtually the whole gamut of mental health subpopulations.

By definition the nurse therapist is someone who effects *therapeutic* change in patients: i.e. assists them to change for the better. Despite this assumption there is a paucity of research evidence to support the view that all nurse therapists are therapeutic, or that this model of care is in any way widespread. Although formal published evidence may be lacking, the philosophy of evaluative research, as described in Chapter 1, is embedded firmly in the practice of behaviour therapy nursing. The approach emphasises the identification of discrete 'patient needs'; the design of appropriate strategies to meet such needs;

and an evaluation of the outcome of the programme of therapy. As noted earlier, writers such as Altschul have asserted that nurses in the United Kingdom have a long history of therapeutic caring for the mentally ill or handicapped person. Until recently there has been little evidence to support this view. Behaviour therapy nursing, which favours the collection of quantitative data to describe the patient's initial presentation and any subsequent changes in the patient's state, has made a contribution to the evaluation of the therapeutic potential of these nurses in particular, and to nurses in general. It should not be forgotten, however, that other kinds of 'nurse therapist' are evident in contemporary practice, and their numbers might be expected to grow in the future. Since such nurses operate within a different theoretical model and, more importantly, hold quite different views about the value of quantitative evaluation, their roles will not be considered here.[1]

(b) The process of nursing

Relations between behaviour therapy nursing and mainstream nursing practice have been strengthened by the emergence of the nursing process (see Ward, 1985). The nursing process emphasises the use of 'scientific method' in clinical practice: collecting assessment data; forming hypotheses about care needs; planning and introducing a specific nursing intervention (or 'care plan'); and evaluating the outcome of this action. This model has been supported at the highest level in Britain since the mid-1970s, when it was argued that nursing was primarily a 'situational activity centred upon goals for living rather than upon a disease/illness concept alone' (SNNMCC, 1976). Authority figures such as Altschul have expressed grave doubts about the value of a 'person-centred', rather than systems or social process model of care (Altschul, 1977, 1978). More recently (1985) she has noted that psychiatric nursing is 'about helping people to increase their ability to exercise their own judgement and [to increase] their ability to cope'. This statement may or may not be a challenge to her earlier views. What is clear is that despite her reservations regarding the process, she has no doubt that the best examples of the nursing process in psychiatric nursing are to be found in the work of the nurse behaviour therapist, where the process is seen 'par excellence'

(Altschul, 1984). Some interesting questions arise from the relationship between a clinical nursing specialty, like behaviour therapy nursing, and mainstream practice. For instance: Is there a common methodological framework? Are all nurses aiming for the same goals as those articulated by Altschul? Are the two streams of clinical practice different in any way? Any answer to these questions must begin with an examination of the work of the nurse therapist. What do such nurses do, and what is their relationship to predominant clinical practice? In the next section of this chapter these questions will be examined by looking at the available published literature on the work and training of the nurse behaviour therapist.

(c) **History**

The earliest report of nurses working within a behavioural model of care was made by Ayllon and Michael (1959). These two psychologists described how nurses in an American state hospital were trained to modify their interactions with psychotic patients in an attempt to reduce the frequency of certain discrete disruptive behaviours (viz. delusional speech, hoarding rubbish, aggression and eating problems). Almost a decade later Gelfand, Gelfand and Dobson (1967) described how anti-therapeutic were the interactions of psychiatric nurses with disturbed patients. This study questioned the validity of traditional dynamic psychotherapy as a framework for nurse–patient interaction. These two studies reflect a kind of turning point in psychiatric and mental handicap nursing. They challenged the assumption that 'care' was always beneficial for the patient. More importantly, they introduced an alternative framework for the study and delivery of care: one which provided an empirical platform for planning and evaluating discrete interactions between the patient and the care-giver. The end of the 1960s saw the beginning of a growing literature on this evaluation of the relationship between nurses and their patients in the mental health sector. Two American studies serve as outstanding examples of the early projection of the aims of behaviour therapy nursing and the methodology of evaluative research. Cockrill and Bernal (1968) designed and evaluated a programme designed to promote verbal behaviour in a withdrawn patient, where reinforcement was provided by a fellow

167

patient. In the same year Peterson and Peterson mounted a complex study in which a package of reinforcement techniques was used in an attempt to control speech, incontinence and self-injury in a severely mentally handicapped child. Cockrill and Bernal's study was one of the first reports of an evaluation of nurses' work where a reversal design (ABAB) was used to evaluate the effects of reinforcement upon the patient's behaviour. The Peterson study used a more complex variant of this single-case experimental design. In their study baseline data were collected (phase A) before introducing the first reinforcement condition (B). A second reinforcement condition was then introduced (C), after which the study reverted to the baseline condition again (A). The study was completed by reinstituting the second reinforcement condition (C) to complete the overall experimental design of A–B–C–A–C.

In Britain the behaviour therapy nursing literature did not emerge until the early 1970s. The earliest reports are in marked contrast to the rigorous, research-based studies of the late 1960s American scene, and are often characterised by a candid acknowledgement of the absence of any serious evaluation of outcome. For instance, in a report on a token economy programme Gray (1972) noted that 'the assessment (evaluation) is a personal observation, and I have kept no behavioural charts'. Over the succeeding 12 years the emphasis on evaluative research has changed, largely in keeping with the growth of nursing research in general. However, as far as the published behaviour therapy literature is concerned, no consistent emphasis upon objective evaluation appears to have been established.

(d) The major targets

This emphasis is much in evidence in the nursing journals which are read widely. A review of the two key British nursing journals (*Nursing Times* and *Nursing Mirror*) shows that 137 articles on behaviour therapy nursing were published between 1970 and 1985 (inclusive). The distribution of articles across 12 main categories is shown in Figure 9.1. Descriptions of the use of behavioural approaches with psychiatric patients, or descriptions of the techniques themselves, dominate the literature. The role of behaviour change methods with the mentally handicapped population is less evident. However, some reports include work with mentally handicapped children, under the umbrella heading of 'children', thereby adding to the proportion of reports within this category. There are few detailed reports of the role of nurses as behaviour therapists, apart from descriptions of the outcome of their interactions with patients. There is also little mention made of their training. There is also a poor representation of reports on assessment and ethical issues, which is a significant weakness given their crucial role in the presentation of care. The publication rate of these articles appears to have been accelerated by the 'nurse as therapist' series which appeared in 1973. This heralded not only more widespread recognition of the potential of the behavioural model of care but also the first description of a formal training programme for nurse therapists (Marks, 1973). The frequency with which such behaviour therapy nursing reports have appeared over the succeeding 12 years has varied between five and 15 articles per annum in these journals. The trend towards publication of such reports appeared to decline towards the end of the 1970s, picking up again in the early 1980s, perhaps as a function of a generalisation of interest in the process of nursing.

Figure 9.1: Distribution of published reports in the *Nursing Times* and *Nursing Mirror* during the period 1970–85

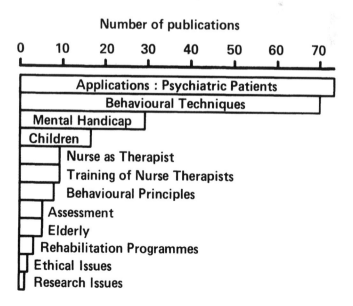

The range of topics which comprise this list of articles is shown in Table 9.1. The focus on psychiatric problems appears to favour evaluations of work with 'neurotic' patients. Specific phobias (Blakey and Greig, 1977), various anxiety states (Brooker, 1980), obsessional behaviour (Eveleigh, 1977) and sexual problems (Simpson, 1982) are classic behaviour therapy targets. In recent years the net has been cast more widely to include eating disorders (Savage and Biley, 1984), health-related anxieties (Sawyer, 1983) and depression (Barker, Hume and Robertson, 1985). In the case where the patient suffers from psychotic or more chronic disorders the topic of the evaluations appears to be more limited in scope: independence training (Brookes and Brown, 1981); speech and social interaction

Table 9.1: Examples of key targets from the nursing literature

Mental handicap

Disturbed behaviour: Pickstock and Taylor (1976); Orton (1979); Birchmore and Claque (1983)
Self-injury: Comley (1976); Barker and Hunter (1977); Slater (1982)
Rocking; Sewpaul *et al.* (1982)
Eating: Pope and Buck (1982); Bushby (1980)
Dressing: Moore and Carr (1976); Patrick and Rafferty (1978)
Speech: Docherty (1978)
Shouting: Birchmore and Claque (1983)
Hyperkinesis: Orton (1979)
Incontinence: Patrick and Rafferty (1978); Orton (1979)

Psychiatric rehabilitation

Independence training: Gray (1972); Brookes and Brown (1981); Chapman (1983); Smith (1984)
Speech: Cliffe (1974); Broome and Collis (1976)
Anti-social behaviour: Seidel and Hodgkinson (1979)

Acute psychiatry

Agoraphobia: Allen (1981)
Anxiety: Brooker (1980)
Phobias: Williamson (1974)
Specific phobias: Blakey and Greig (1977); Sawyer (1983)
Obsessional behaviour: Eveleigh (1977); Farrington (1983); Mercer (1984)
Sexual dysfunction: Simpson (1982)
Bulimia: Savage and Biley (1984)
Depression: Barker, Hume and Robertson (1985)
Child abuse: Gilbert (1976); Manchester (1981)

The elderly

Confusion: Merchant and Saxby (1981)
Sleep: Burton and Spall (1981)
Activity: Burton and Spall (1981); Joyce and Dustin (1982)
Incontinence: Linke (1982)

(Cliffe, 1974) and specific behavioural problems (Seidel and Hodgkinson, 1979). A similar picture is reflected in the mental handicap reports. A wide range of programmes have been described which tackle more serious patterns of disturbed behaviour: self-injury (Barker and Hunter, 1977) or self-stimulation (Sewpaul, Thorpe and Tyerman, 1982). Most of the other reports have focused upon self-care or social skills training. However, these targets occur often against a background of some form of disturbed behaviour (e.g. Patrick and Rafferty, 1978; Bushby, 1980). Reports involving the elderly are few in number and tend to focus on the maintenance of socially appropriate behaviour in the institutional setting. There are also reports of work with confused elderly people (Merchant and Saxby, 1981) and incontinence (Linke, 1982), both of which are crucial targets in this area of nursing. As noted earlier there have been very few reports of the training of nurses in behavioural methods within these two journals. Most reports are anecdotal in nature or describe only the framework of the training. The most rigorous evaluations of this area of interest have been reported in other journals which emphasise research (e.g. Milne, Burdett and Conway, 1985) or which are devoted exclusively to behaviour therapy (e.g. Woods and Cullen, 1983). The focus of the reports illustrated above is fairly specific. Most ask the question, 'to what extent is it possible to resolve problematic patterns of behaviour by use of a behavioural model of care?' As we shall discover shortly, some of these reports try to answer this question by rigorous evaluation, whereas others are more casual in their approach. The same aims appear to be evident in the staff training literature. Most purport to train nurses in specific skills or methods of intervention, but often fail to report any serious evaluation of how this is achieved, if at all.

(e) The evaluation methods

There are a wide range of evaluation methods used in the reports referred to above. It might be reasonable to assume that as nurses became more sophisticated the 'soft evaluations' favoured by some of the early writers would be replaced by tighter methods of critical evaluation, where both method and outcome were subjected to closer analysis. As the following

171

review illustrates, this does not appear to be the case. Five main categories of evaluation have been used. These are as follows:

1. Clinical impressions

In this category no objective data are presented. Instead, the views, or judgements, of the participating staff are reported. Gray's (1972) report mentioned earlier is an example of this kind of subjective evaluation. A similar anecdotal account of a token economy programme was published much more recently (Chapman, 1983). This type of evaluation is not the exclusive preserve of the 'unsophisticated' or novice writer. In a recent evaluation of a clinical project in which a nurse collaborated with very senior medical staff, clinical impressions figured strongly in the outcome evaluation of the project (Goldberg, Bridges, Cooper et al., 1985).

2. Global ratings

A general evaluation of the patient's progress is possible through use of some kind of rating scale which covers a wide range of target areas. Clarke (1983) used a specially designed 'adaptive behaviour scale' to evaluate change in overall functioning in hospitalised patients; and Brookes and Brown (1981) used a similar format to evaluate change in target behaviours for patients within a rehabilitation programme.

3. Specific ratings

A more specific evaluation is possible through use of a rating scale which provides a measure of a specific target area. For example Cliffe (1974) described the rating of the amount of speech uttered by withdrawn patients; Eveleigh (1977) rated the amount of avoidance behaviour shown by the patient; and Sawyer (1983) assessed the amount of change in reported fear. The common thread for all these ratings is that they were completed by staff, based upon their actual observation of the patient.

4. Self-report ratings

This class of evaluation differs from (3) above in that they are completed by the patients themselves, although staff may provide varying degrees of assistance in their completion. Williamson (1974) asked patients who were described as agoraphobic to rate their 'freedom from fear' on completion of a therapeutic project; Gilbert (1976) asked mothers to rate the extent to which they enjoyed contact with their child; Brooker (1980) asked patients to rate their levels of anxiety across various everyday situations; and Mercer (1984) asked depressed patients to monitor their mood level using this kind of self-report format.

5. Direct observation

This final category embraces a wide range of discrete measures of the actual behaviour of the patient. Frequency measures have proven to be the most popular: how often does the patient engage in specific self-injurious behaviour? (Barker and Hunter, 1977); how often does he ask to visit the toilet? (Patrick and Rafferty, 1978); how often does he speak in an audible voice as opposed to a whisper? (Docherty, 1978); or how often does he pull his hair out or try to abscond from the hospital? (Orton, 1979). In some cases the frequency of occurrence of an observed behaviour is presented as a percentage of the total behaviour observed (Barker, 1976). However, in most cases the data are presented as a simple 'tally count' of the target behaviour. Where the behaviour is of variable duration the length of time the patient spends engaged in the behaviour may be measured. In some cases this may be calculated as a percentage of the total observation time: e.g. time spent rocking (Sewpaul *et al.*, 1982) or the time spent engaged in various social behaviours (Joyce and Dustin, 1982). Some reports specify the actual time spent in the behaviour: e.g. time spent sitting dressed (Patrick and Rafferty, 1978); time spent sleeping (Burton and Spall, 1981); or time spent shouting (Birchmore and Claque, 1983). Within this direct observation category I would include also measures of the administration of medication (Broome and Collis, 1976; Pickstock and Taylor, 1976) and the measurement of the patient's weight (Savage and Biley, 1984).

(f) General comment

This brief review is limited to the extent that it focuses attention exclusively upon two British nursing journals. Why did I not consider the literature from the United States where behaviour therapy nursing found its roots? My reason for this is as follows. Firstly, the concept of the nurse specialist in behaviour therapy is largely a British phenomenon. It seemed correct, therefore, to review the British nursing literature which served as a background to this development. Secondly, a review of the *International Nursing Index* for the past 15 years suggests that the frequency of reports on behaviour therapy nursing is higher in British journals than in similar American publications. Reports in these other journals cover very similar territory to those targets already cited: anxiety management (Tamez, Moore and Brown, 1978); eating disorders (Schmidt and Duncan, 1974; Claggett, 1980); disturbed behaviour in institutions (O'Brien, Caldwell and Transeau, 1985) and care of the elderly (Prehn, 1982). It would appear, also, that the nature and quality of the evaluations of these clinical projects does not differ widely from those already reviewed in the British literature.

(g) Evaluation illustrations

A distinction can also be drawn between those studies where a specific method of evaluation is used to assess change in only one area of functioning, and those reports where a range of evaluations may be used across several target areas. Barker and Hunter's single-case study of self-injury would illustrate the former whilst Sawyer's multifaceted study of a cancer phobic is a good illustration of the latter. Some reports have also tried to discuss the evaluation of projects from more than one angle; perhaps in an attempt to answer more than one question. For instance Barker (1976) reported a study which attempted to reduce levels of self-stimulatory behaviour shown by four profoundly mentally handicapped men. Staff completed ratings of each patient's behaviour (a specific rating); measures were taken of the frequency of occurrence of certain target behaviours (direct observation); notes were made of the extent to which the group walked around and sat at the meal table (clinical impressions); discrete measures of the amount of tranquillising medication given to the patients during the project were recorded (direct observation); a record was made of the use of mechanical restraint in hours and minutes each day (direct observation); and staff reported on perceived levels of social interaction within the group (clinical impressions). As a result, the 'outcome' of the project was evaluated in terms of changes in the target behaviours, supported by evaluations of changes in social interaction, ambulation, table etiquette and need for control by drugs or physical restraint.

In some of these reports the time scale of the projects is relatively short. In the study referred to above the project spanned 6 months exactly. A question could be raised here about the validity of an evaluation within such a short time scale. How significant is the change which occurs over so short a period of time, especially when the patient has been hospitalised for many years? It could be argued that where the patient has been 'chronic' for many years, any change achieved within a short period of time is highly significant. Of greater importance is the question 'does the observed change last?' The study involving the four men described briefly above is most deficient in this respect, in that it included no long-term follow-up measures. We have no way of knowing, therefore, whether or not the change which occurred was maintained after the project was completed. In contrast to this situation, the report by Barker, Docherty, Hird and Hunter (1978) described a study of a group of mentally handicapped children who were involved in a large-scale self-care and social skills training programme. The study reported upon gains made during the active phase of the programme, and included a 4-month follow-up evaluation. This evaluation was designed to assess the degree to which perform- ance decreased following the discontinuation of the active reinforcement phase.

In a slightly different vein other reports have evaluated the patient's behaviour across situations other than the original 'treatment' setting. For instance, Docherty (1978) measured the number of times an adolescent with Down's syndrome spoke in a whisper or audibly across three different situations within his ward environment. Moore and Carr (1976) counted the number of garments which a severely mentally handicapped child put on correctly under different conditions, and when handed the clothing in a certain order. This project aimed to assess the advantages, if any, of a systematic training programme over more conventional means of training. It is also possible to evaluate the effect upon the patient's behaviour of different treatment conditions, or modifications to the primary inter- vention strategy. An example of this kind of evaluation is found in Barker and Hunter's (1977) evaluation of a programme aimed at reducing minor self-injury in a severely mentally handicapped child. A measure of the frequency of skin-picking was taken within a certain time period as a baseline. The same measure was employed during the treatment stages, up to and including a 4-month follow-up. The frequency of skin-picking was studied as a number of reinforcement conditions were implemented in succession. This case illustrates the use of an extension of the basic A–B design referred to earlier (see Hersen and Barlow, 1976, Chapter 6 for a discussion). Finally, the evaluation can be extended to include a much longer-term assessment of outcome. Sawyer (1983), for instance, helped a cancer phobic patient to rate certain fears (viz. the development of cancer and death) as well as rating the overall *severity* of her handicap; staying alone in the house; the degree of discomfort when bathing her breasts; visiting the crematorium and wearing her dead mother's ring and watch. These self-report measures formed the basis for an evaluation of change during therapy and were repeated at intervals of 4, 6, 9 and 13 weeks; and later at a 5- and 9-month follow-up.

Can we make any general observations about these reports from the behaviour therapy nursing literature? It is clear that the aims of the evaluations vary greatly. In some cases the intention is to assess the extent to which certain interventions produce change in specific areas of the patient's functioning. In others an attempt is made to judge the value of nursing care in more global terms: is the patient more independent? is he more capable of facing difficult situations? An example of this latter broader focus can be found in a report by Tilley (1985). The patient was treated for multiple phobias and rejected offers of help with a bereavement reaction. Tilley suggested, however, that there was some evidence that the patient's pathological grief diminished as a result of exposure to treatment for related phobic problems. In some of the reports an attempt is made to judge whether or not short-term change is maintained by the inclusion of follow-up evaluation measures. On a similar plane some studies investigate whether or not changes which occur under one set of conditions will 'generalise' to other settings within the patient's environment. This generalisation issue is in evidence in some of the staff training studies, where it is important to find out if change in knowledge or skill, which is shown in the classroom, also occurs in the clinical situation and is maintained beyond the active phase of the teaching programme. Milne's (1984) study of the extent to which nurses' behaviour on the ward changed as a result of participation in a classroom-based programme is a fine example of just such an evaluation. Within these various reports can also be found other interesting outcome evaluations which are of a more 'distal' nature. What savings might be made on medication charges as a result of a behavioural management programme (Barker, 1976)? What savings on laundry services might result from an incontinence reduction programme (Hartie and Black, 1975)?

Besides the aims of these studies, variations are evident also in the methods used to answer such questions. Some studies employ only anecdotal accounts which, on their own, may be of suspect validity. As noted earlier, however, this is not a problem which is exclusive to nursing. Only a small proportion of the studies reported here used objective means of data collection, such as direct observation. More importantly, even where such observations were used there is rarely any account of the reliability of these observations. Bushby (1980) is one of the few exceptions which reported on the method used to calculate the reliability of the different observers involved in the collection of the data. It was noted earlier that the American reports of the late 1960s included the use of specific research designs to evaluate change in the patient's performance. In general there has been little use made of single-case study methodology in the British literature. Barker's use of multiple baseline design across *subjects* in a study of nocturnal enuresis (1979), and his use of multiple baseline across various self-care and social *behaviours* within a token economy system (1980) appear to be two of the few exceptions to this rule. In general the nature of evaluation used appears to be strongly related to the training the nurses had received. For instance, nurses who have experienced the behavioural psychotherapy training begun at the Maudsley Hospital in the early 1970s tend to favour evaluations which rely upon therapist's, or patient's self-report, ratings. Those nurses who have worked within a behaviour analysis framework appear to favour the use of more direct evaluations of the patient's behaviour.

9.2 EVALUATING PRACTICE: TWO ILLUSTRATIONS

From this brief review it should be apparent that behaviour therapy nursing, as a definable activity, is possessed of an erratic and inconsistent history. In this section I want to consider the

177

kind of evaluative questions which might be asked to help clarify our understanding of this aspect of service delivery. First of all there would appear to be a need to evaluate the skills which nurses acquire in training programmes. We need also to ask how these skills generalise to the clinical arena. Such a training effect has been studied carefully in some highly specific programmes (cf. Marks *et al.*, 1977). However, where nurses are trained to work with a broader patient population, or within a less delimited model of therapy, this question has received only cursory attention. Some consideration will be given to this question here. Secondly, there appears to be a need to describe the role of the 'nurse as therapist' in more detail. As we have noted already, a wide range of nurses, from a range of backgrounds, working with an equally wide range of patients, have described their work as being within a behavioural framework of care. However, it is clear that the concept of the 'nurse therapist' is associated with a far more limited role, within a highly select nursing population. Given that a number of different training programmes are now in operation, producing different kinds of 'nurse therapist', there may be a need to evaluate the kinds of roles these nurses have developed, in relation to different clinical groups. This consideration will be addressed in the second part of this section.

(a) The evaluation of clinical performance

The aims of the Scottish National Board training programme in behaviour therapy nursing are threefold. Firstly there is the emphasis upon the acquisition of knowledge, evaluated by the student's ability to answer specific questions orally or in written form. Secondly there is an evaluation of the student's ability to translate these principles into practice, tested by such means as the selection of appropriate methods in the assessment or design of a care programme. Finally, there is an emphasis upon the acquisition of discrete skills, involving the practice of certain methods of assessment or behaviour change. These are evaluated by direct observation of the student. A commonplace criticism of many educational programmes is that they do not emphasise the acquisition of the skills necessary for the job. Such is the emphasis given to written examinations in basic nurse training that it would appear that nurses are prepared for writing and thinking, rather than for actually practising the art. Over the past decade the behaviour therapy nursing course in Dundee has tried to develop measures which will provide a satisfactory measure of the student's practical problem-solving and clinical skills. In this section I shall discuss briefly the format used by the clinical supervisor to evaluate the student's performance in the management of each clinical project undertaken during training. Given that equal standards of difficulty could not be arranged for each student, there is no absolute requirement for the student to be successful in his/her intervention. Instead, the evaluation measures the extent to which the student used the skills and knowledge acquired by that stage of his/her training, in the therapeutic exercise.

The format

The format under discussion here is illustrated in Figure 9.2. The present format has been developed from three earlier versions, used with small classes of students ($N=6$). Each class of student has worked with a broad range of client groups: children and adults with a mental handicap, in hospital and the community; adults with acute and more chronic forms of psychiatric disorder; and elderly people with psychological problems. The format is still under review in terms of its reliability.

A process measure

The format evaluates the critical features of the therapeutic programme, irrespective of the situation in which the programme is mounted, or the client group who represent the target of the programme. Therefore the format can be used to evaluate the student's direct individual contact with a single patient or his contact with a group of patients through the medium of staff who are involved in running the clinical project. The format deals with the 'process' of therapy, including the student's relationship with the patient or significant others; his/her ability to organise the various stages of the programme; his/her ability to identify and solve problems met at any stage in the process; as well as his/her use and understanding of the various 'technical' aspects of the implementation of the programme. Although not essential, the format also includes an evaluation of the student's ability to describe the development and outcome of the programme in the form of a clinical report. These various skills and judgements are thought to represent the construct of 'good clinical practice'.

The supervisor

Each student is allocated to a number of supervisors, each of whom is responsible for monitoring all aspects of the case, from initial contact through to final report. Each case is discussed once a week using the format as the basis for this discussion. The student is asked to report progress to date, explaining the selection of goals, use or adaptation of specific methods and related issues concerning the organisation of the programme. The student's understanding of the role and action of the methods selected and used is evaluated most closely during the assessment and programme planning phases. In addition to this indirect evaluation, the supervisor may also study any materials used in the programme: completed assessment charts; visual aids designed for staff or patient use; graphs and other summary charts; and progress notes. The supervisor may accompany the student on selected sessions to evaluate performance in the clinical area. Alternatively, the supervisor may ask the student to record sessions on audio- or video-tape, if this is more appropriate. These evaluation sessions are determined by the supervisor and are arranged at intervals to obtain measures of the student's performance at critical stages in the development of the therapeutic programme.

The rating method

Each supervisor is supplied with guidelines which illustrate a scale for use with each item on the format. The student's performance is evaluated using a five-point rating: 1 representing the lowest standard — 'poor or unacceptable'; 5 representing the highest standard — 'excellent or very acceptable'. The mid-point rating (3) represents the minimum acceptable standard of skill execution or understanding with '2' and '4' representing below and above this minimum standard, respectively.

This format was developed to evaluate the trainee nurse behaviour therapist's performance across a range of 'practice skills'. The ratings are based upon *direct observation* of the student's interaction with the patient or his/her significant others, or observation of a recording of this interaction if more appropriate. The student's *oral responses*, elicited during super-

Figure 9.2: The clinical experience record

BEHAVIOUR THERAPY NURSING COURSE
CLINICAL EXPERIENCE RECORD

STUDENTS NAME .... OPTION ....

DATE OF ASSESSMENT .... ASSESSMENT No .... SIGNAT. ....

A GENERAL	RATING	COMMENTS
1. Relationship with patient		
2. Relationship with sig. others		
3. Organisation		
4. Problem-solving		
5. EFFORT		

B ASSESSMENT	RATING	COMMENTS
1. Selection		
2. Handling		
3. Guidelines		
4. Rationale		
5. Expectations/Orientation		

C TREATMENT PLAN	RATING	COMMENTS
1. Identification of final targets		
2. Identification of sub-targets		
3. Guidelines		
4. Rationale		
5. Technique selection		
6. Selection of recording method (s)		

D TREATMENT PROGRESS	RATING	COMMENTS
1. Structure/Organisation		
2. Implementation		
3. Evaluation		
4. Adaptation/Modification		

E REPORTING	RATING	COMMENTS
1. Content		
2. Style		
3. Presentation		

I have read the above and have discussed this with my supervisor.

Signed .... Date ....

vision sessions, are included in this evaluation, as are any significant *permanent products* associated with the design or implementation of the programme. These ratings are used as a supplement to evaluations of 'learning' in the classroom, where tests of knowledge and the student's ability to replicate specific techniques which have been modelled during training are also

181

undertaken. Given that these classroom tests evaluate the skills and knowledge base acquired in the training area (the classroom itself) the rating format could be seen as a generalisation measure: to what extent does the student 'carry over' skills and knowledge from the classroom to the clinical area?

The rating has a dual function. It is used, first of all, to provide feedback to the student on his performance to date in the clinical training programme. The student studies the ratings given and comments made, before discussing these with the supervisor. The ratings may reinforce the student's awareness of specific areas of competence or deficit, or may serve to draw attention to areas of functioning which require consolidation or development. This allows each student to be monitored closely, by a range of supervisors, identifying at the earliest opportunity any problems in skill uptake or usage, and providing a forum for resolving these problems. The format also allows the evaluation of competence and the reinforcement of positive performance as appropriate.

The second function of the format involves the evaluation of the 'training effect'. In the classroom each student is assessed at intervals in terms of the acquisition of specific skills and their underlying concepts. These evaluations are conducted in the form of an oral examination with, where appropriate, a request to 'demonstrate' a specific skill. Under these examination conditions it is possible to rate the student's use of specific skills and his/her knowledge of their rationale. In the clinical setting the task facing the student is more complex. Here the student is required to exercise judgement regarding the selection of strategies of assessment or intervention; and may need to use a number of different skills in a 'therapeutic package'. In this context it appears more appropriate to evaluate the student's approach to the patient overall, providing a rating of his/her overall usage of certain methods or concepts. If the classroom ratings and tests evaluate the student's ability to learn discrete skills under controlled conditions, the format described may be seen as evaluating his/her deployment of these skills and concepts under the less stable conditions of the clinical setting.

It should be emphasised that the format described is still under review and additional data are required before its reliability can be determined. Furthermore, the format has not been evaluated outwith the confines of the Dundee course. As a result we are unable to evaluate the efficiency of the operational guidelines which are used to assist the supervisor's ratings, given that there are other venues at which supervisors can discuss the rating and compare notes. However, despite these reservations the format described does appear to offer an additional insight into the training of nurses as behaviour therapists. The format appears to offer supervisors a structure for evaluating the student's organisation of the programme, use of the therapist–patient relationship, and selection and usage of specific therapeutic skills. Providing that the supervisor is sensitive to the needs of the patient, the format can be used to evaluate the generalisation of 'practice skills' across a wide range of client groups.

(b) The evaluation of the nurse therapist's role

Mention has already been made of the paucity of information on the outcome of training nurses as behaviour therapists. The seminal study by Marks and his colleagues led to an evaluation of the 'therapeutic outcome' of the training programme: to what extent did the nurses help their patients? Their conclusion was that these nurses were at least as successful as psychologists and psychiatrists when treating mainly phobic patients using similar methods. This study has been criticised by Milne (1986) on the grounds that it provides no real evaluation of the training programme's effects on the nurse's subsequent role as therapist. Thus, although this study represents a measure of the effectiveness of the nurse therapists, the absence of baseline measures and information about the skills and knowledge offered by the course does not allow us to attribute the nurses' efficacy to the training programme itself.

It has also been noted that the Maudsley training model is an ill-fitting one for the nurse therapist in general, given its limited focus on 'adult neurotics'. The behaviour therapy nursing course, which is based upon the Dundee psychiatric services, has, over the past decade, tried to break the mould of the 'nurse therapist' by emphasising the potential of a behavioural approach at a number of levels of sophistication, across a range of client groups (see Barker, Ellis and Hunt, 1985). A number of questions need to be asked about such a training course. What kind of nurses are produced and what kind of roles do they play? With what kind of people, and with what sort of problems, do they deal? What aspects of the training programme do they incorporate into their work and what developments in their careers occur as a result of exposure to the programme of training? An attempt was made to begin such an evaluation in 1978, when 20 nurses had progressed through the programme (see Barker, 1980). A subsequent follow-up study was mounted using a similar method in 1982 and a retrospective study of all 64 nurses who had completed training by the summer of 1984 was completed in 1985. In this section I wish to discuss some of the findings of this latter study.

The survey

Data were collected by a postal questionnaire circulated to all nurses who had completed the training at least 6 months prior to the beginning of the survey. The former students were asked to complete a 14-page multiple-choice questionnaire, which also provided space for more open-ended replies, subsequently coded. As Figure 9.3 shows, only three nurses were untraced: of the 61 contacted over half were working in a 'nurse behaviour therapist' role of some description. Eight nurses admitted that they were not practising the skills offered by their training to any significant degree. A further five nurses had left the service. Eleven nurses had been promoted to senior nurse positions. Eight of these, including one director and three assistant direc-

Figure 9.3: Roles of former behaviour therapy nursing students on follow-up, 1976–84 (N=64)

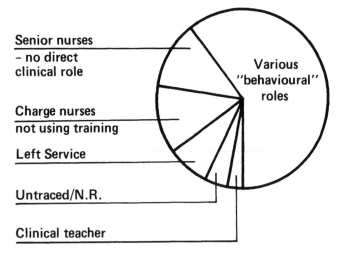

Senior nurses
– no direct
clinical role

Charge nurses
not using training

Left Service

Untraced/N.R.

Clinical teacher

Various "behavioural" roles

tors of nursing services, had no direct clinical contact with patients, but believed that the training was of relevance to their present work. The remaining three senior nurses all maintained a substantial clinical caseload as part of their work. Only one nurse had moved into the educational field following training.

Figure 9.4 shows how these career developments correlate with the 12 courses mounted between 1976 and 1984. The shaded and black areas represent the 40 nurses involved in behaviour therapy nursing on a largely full-time basis. As the figure shows, the proportion of nurses who have moved into 'nurse specialist' posts has increased over the past 5 years. The figure also shows that six of the eight nurses 'not practising' came from the first 5 years of the course, as also did three of the nurses who left the service and the three who were lost from the follow-up. Although this 'drop-out' rate may be explained in terms of the passage of time, the increased demand for places, plus the pressure on funding, may have changed the nature of students admitted to the course in recent years.

Forty nurses were involved in the delivery of a clinical

Figure 9.4: Summary of roles in terms of year of training

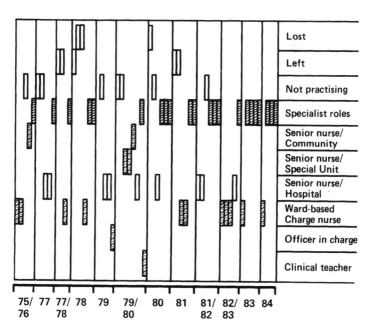

behavioural service of one form or another (62.5 per cent of the total sample: 71.4 per cent of the nurses traced and still within the service). Approximately two-thirds of these nurses represented psychiatry, the rest were from mental handicap: this reflects the proportion of training places available for each speciality. The mental handicap nurses were evenly divided between those working in a special 'behavioural ward' setting, and those who were 'nurse specialists': i.e. offering advice and training to their colleagues on the planning and management of a behavioural nursing service for a unit or whole hospital. In psychiatry less than half the nurses offered a service to *either* the rehabilitation area *or* the acute sector alone. More than half of the psychiatric nurses worked as 'nurse specialists' offering a direct therapeutic and consultative service to the whole psychiatric service, rather than specific sub-populations.

Targets and methods

In the survey published in 1980 details were reported of the kinds of methods used by the nurses in their dealings with various patient groups. In the more recent study an attempt was made to repeat this detailed survey with the much larger sample. However, the detail which emerged appeared to obscure the picture. Here I have simplified the results greatly in order to gain a clearer idea of what sort of approaches were favoured by the nurses.

The most popular methods of the group as a whole were those involving prompting, modelling, reinforcement techniques and anxiety management. Seventy-five per cent of the sample reported use of these techniques. The open-ended replies showed that many nurses acknowledged the importance of reinforcement and modelling as the basis of most nurse–therapist interactions, whether in the acute or the long-stay sector. It was also interesting to note that many nurses in the mental handicap field reported using modified anxiety management methods with institutionalised patients. Skills training methods — which ranged from basic self-help skills training through to the acquisition of sophisticated interpersonal skills — were the next most popular intervention. Although important information is lost by bringing all such methods together under one broad heading, it is clear that the 'constructional approach' reflected by skills training is an important part of the nurse's armamentarium. It is also worth noting that punishment methods and response prevention, two approaches which are part of traditional behaviour therapy, were used only to a limited extent by this sample. Taking their place, to a great extent, may be the various methods embraced by 'cognitive therapy' an approach which has received increasing attention in the teaching programme over the past 5 years.

Figure 9.5: Former students' use of therapeutic methods

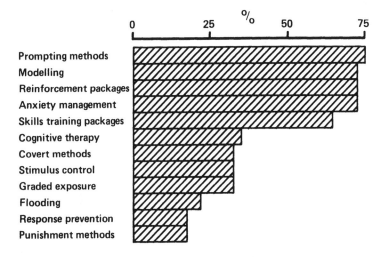

Figure 9.6 illustrates the distribution of attention paid to various clinical problems, through individual and group therapy. By far the most popular area of clinical interest was social skills deficit tackled on a group basis. More than 80 per cent of the sample reported dealing with *basic* social skills deficits by this approach. It is interesting to note that less than 30 per cent of the sample reported dealing with more advanced *interpersonal* skills deficit; i.e. assertiveness, anger management, etc. Social skills deficits were tackled both in the acute and the long-stay hospital population, and may reflect a traditional area of focus for nursing intervention. As might be expected, anxiety and phobic disorders occupy a high position on the overall table. It is interesting, however, that *generalised* anxiety should be slightly more common a target area than phobic disorders. Self-care and domestic skills training were widely dealt with in group rehabilitation programmes. Other institutional problems, such as aggression and self-injury, were more often tackled on an

Figure 9.6: Proportion of former students engaged in work with different problem areas. Shaded columns indicate group work; clear columns represent work with individuals

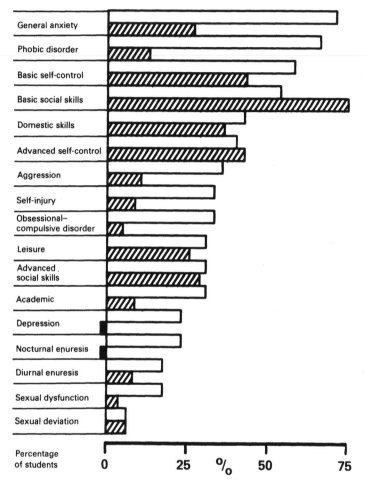

individual basis. Depression represents a significant entry into this chart: in 1980 it was not reported at all. In 1984 approximately 20 per cent of the sample reported dealing with this problem. The relatively low level of attention paid to sexual problems may reflect the specialist nature of sexual problems which in many areas, such as Dundee, inhabit only the fringes of the mental health field.

In addition to the clinical categories indicated, former students added further information about other problems with which they dealt. Most prominent in this additional area were drug dependence (specifically tranquillisers); bulimia; pain management; pre-menstrual syndrome; and public-speaking anxiety. These problems were represented uniquely in the community setting. For the hospitalised populations the nurses picked out aggression, destructiveness and motivational deficit in the mental handicap area and various problems associated with gross psychosis in long-stay psychiatry.

General use of training

The students were also asked a number of general questions about their general 'role'. Almost 70 per cent of the sample thought that they used their training as much as was appropriate for the area in which they worked; 12 per cent believing that they could devote some more time to behaviour therapy; and 20 per cent expressing the view that their training was much underused. Reasons given for the dissatisfaction expressed by this third of the sample ranged from staff shortages for those working in hospital settings, to the resistance of senior staff colleagues who did not support this model of care. In all settings 'other commitments', such as routine administration, supervision of learners, meetings, etc., were seen as a major obstacle to the fulfilment of their role. Overall, the majority of the sample believed that they had been well trained to carry out their present roles: 56 per cent felt that they had been 'very well prepared' and 34 per cent 'quite well prepared'.

Comment

The Scottish National Board's training programme in behaviour therapy nursing is unique in that it offers training to nurses from disparate backgrounds within the same course. By ignoring the traditional boundaries (e.g. between 'neurotic', 'psychotic' and 'mentally handicapped' people) it has shown an attempt to align itself to the radical behavioural notion that the person's behaviour represents his major problem of living. With nurses from different clinical backgrounds trying to share the same model of patient care, it is not surprising that a slightly different kind of 'nurse therapist' should emerge from the programme. At least three levels of nurse therapist are evident to date: the ward-based clinician who co-ordinates care-planning within a behavioural framework; the independent practitioner working directly with individuals or groups of patients mainly in the community; and the nurse specialist who provides an advisory service to colleagues in addition to the maintenance of a clinical caseload. Although not explained by the data reported here, it is apparent that the variables which determine which nurses adopt which roles are largely unrelated to the training programme itself. The data discussed here do, however, suggest that the majority of nurses trained within this model over the past decade are consolidating their position within the clinical field, and are offering a service which reflects the broad range of clinical problems represented in the literature review.

In summary, the aims of this survey were simple: to find out what happens to nurses on completion of their training; to identify the kind of roles they developed; and to describe the kinds of methods adopted in relation to different clinical problems or situations. There should be no need to emphasise that this evaluation is very much a 'work in progress': data have been collected routinely 6 months after the completion of each course for the past 8 years; the retrospective evaluation described here has been completed twice to date, and will be repeated every 5 years. The picture which emerges from this evaluation, although simple, is important. Detailed information on the actual 'work' of the nurse therapist has been scarce. This survey makes one kind of contribution to the analysis of this facet of mental health nursing provision. The evaluative method does, however, have its deficiencies. The data reflect in the main the student's perception of his/her work, and requires to be treated with the caution reserved for all self-report data. The format of the survey, with its reliance upon structured questions, with accompanying ratings, demanded a rejection of amplifying detail in many instances. Where additional information was supplied, this was coded and categorised, again with a resultant loss of information. However, given that the same format has been in use for almost a decade it is possible to make comparisons across courses, as well as across students and their individual careers. The data are being analysed at present to provide information about the relative length of the students' clinical career following training; the role of the training in the attainment of promotion; the nature of the nurse's clinical role in relation to different clinical populations; and the nurse's role in basic and post-basic education, and in research.

9.3 CONCLUSION

In this chapter I have reviewed some of the literature which reflects the development of the nurse as a behaviour therapist. Over the past 15 years this development has occurred against a background of increasing interest in systematic care-planning and evaluation, expressed through the nursing process movement and nursing research in general. As a result, the activities of the nurse working within a discrete therapeutic model are not as alien now as they were in the early days of the nurse therapist movement. The original British training programme continues to run at the Maudsley Hospital and has been replicated in three other centres to date. Other kinds of training have emerged, such as the Scottish programme noted in this chapter. Most significant of all has been the recognition that many different forms of training are possible within various different clinical settings, to meet different professional 'needs'. The variety of these contributions to service provision and professional career development has been summarised in detail by Milne (1986).

It should not be forgotten that the concept of the nurse as a therapist is hardly a novel one. The first steps towards the establishment of formal nurse therapist status was taken in places such as the Henderson Hospital and Dingleton, where the 'therapeutic community' was first promulgated (see Morrice, 1980). The nurse as a behaviour therapist is of interest not because the concept is a novel one, but because it reflects an interest in the development of the nurse's role based upon the kind of evaluative research reflected in this text. It should not be forgotten that, although for many the nurse therapist is associated with a fairly limited clinical role with an equally limited clinical population, the potential of this model of nursing extends far beyond the boundaries of the mental health setting (see Reavley and Herdman, 1985).

Although behaviour therapy nursing has grown out of a rigorous, empirical–evaluative approach to the study of mental disorder, it is significant that nurse therapists themselves have contributed little to the evaluative literature. I should qualify that by saying that the major research contributions have been made by medical or psychological researchers, with nurses acting in only a supportive role. With the exception of a few studies, most of the reports which furnish valid data on aspects of behaviour therapy nursing are single-case studies. While these can be highly valuable media for the critical evaluation of the outcome of therapy, in many instances information on the reliability and validity of the data is missing. In other cases the absence of a sophisticated experimental design encourages caution in the interpretation of the results. It would be interesting to know whether the many trained nurse behaviour therapists have been unable or disinclined to mount more rigorous evaluations of the many facets of this new face of mental health nursing. As we progress towards the 1990s and nursing research becomes more accepted as a 'routine' activity, one would anticipate that more nurses will begin to collect the kind of data described here. This will be their own contribution to the evaluation and development of the nurse behaviour therapist.

NOTE

1. Hardin and Durham (1985) report a study of nurse therapists in the United States of America, where the respondents appeared to work mainly within family therapy or individual counselling models. The nurse therapists were asked to indicate whether or not they thought they could improve their therapeutic performance through the use of more concrete methods of evaluation. Only 4 per cent of the respondents answered yes.

REFERENCES

Allen, K.W. (1981) 'Behavioural Treatment of an Agoraphobic', *Nursing Times, 77*, pp. 268-70

Altschul, A.T. (1977) 'Use of the Nursing Process in Psychiatric Care', *Nursing Times, 73*, pp. 1412-13

Altschul. A.T. (1978) 'A Systems Approach to the Nursing Process', *Journal of Advanced Nursing, 3*, pp. 333-40

Altschul, A.T. (1984) 'Does Good Practice Need Good Principles?', *Nursing Times, 80*, pp. 49-51

Altschul, A.T. (1985) Introduction, in: P. Barker and D. Fraser (eds), *The Nurse as Therapist: A Behavioural Model*, Croom Helm, London

Ayllon, T. and Michael, J. (1959) 'The Psychiatric Nurse as a Behavioural Engineer', *Journal of the Experimental Analysis of Behaviour, 2*, pp. 323-34

Barker, P. (1976)'Changing Image': The Reduction of Self-stimulatory Behaviour in Four Profoundly Retarded Males', *International Journal of Nursing Studies. 13*, pp. 179-86

Barker, P. (1979) 'Noctural Enuresis: An Experimental Study Involving Two Behavioural Approaches', *International Journal of Nursing Studies*, 16, pp. 319-27

Barker, P. (1980) 'Behaviour Therapy in Psychiatric and Mental Handicap Nursing', *Journal of Advanced Nursing*, 5, pp. 55-69

Barker, P. (1982) *Behaviour Therapy Nursing*, Croom Helm, London

Barker, P. and Hunter, M.H. (1977) 'Minor Self Mutilation', *Nursing Times*, 73, pp. 500-2

Barker, P., Docherty, P., Hird, J. and Hunter, M.H. (1978) 'Living and Learning: A Nurse Administered Token Economy Programme Involving Mentally Handicapped Schoolboys', *International Journal of Nursing Studies*, 15, pp. 91-102

Barker, P., Docherty, P. and Hird, J. (1980) 'Showing an Improvement: An Examination of Variables Central to the Token Economy System', *International Journal of Nursing Studies*, 17, pp. 25-37

Barker, P., Hume, A. and Robertson, W. (1985), 'Psychological Therapy in Affective Disorder', *Nursing Mirror*, 160, pp. 34-6

Barker, P. Ellis, J. and Hunt (1985) 'Behaviour Therapy Nursing: Horses for Courses', *Nursing Times*, 161, pp. 29-31

Birchmore, T. and Claque, S. (1983) 'A Behavioural Approach to Reduce Shouting', *Nursing Times*, 79, pp. 37-9

Blakey, R. and Greig, K. (1977) 'Severe Cat Phobia', *Nursing Times*, 73, pp. 1106-8

Brooker, C. (1980) 'Behavioural Management of a Complex Case', *Nursing Times*, 76, pp. 367-9

Brookes, P.J. and Brown, C. (1981) 'A Behavioural Approach to Psychiatric Rehabilitation', *Nursing Times*, 77, pp. 367-70

Broome, A. and Collis, B. (1976) 'A Patient for Behaviour Modification', *Nursing Times*, 72, pp. 580-81

Burton, M. and Spall, G. (1981) 'The Behavioural Approach to Nursing the Elderly', *Nursing Times*, 77, pp. 247-8

Bushby, S. (1980) 'Training the Mentally Handicapped: The Reinforcers', *Nursing Mirror*, 151, pp. 18-20

Chapman, S. (1983) 'Cash on Delivery', *Nursing Mirror*, 156, pp. 14-15

Claggett, M.S. (1980) 'Anorexia Nervosa: A Behavioral Approach', *American Journal of Nursing*, 80, pp. 1471-2

Clarke, I. (1983) 'The Story of Jane', *Nursing Times*, 79, pp. 33-5

Cliffe, M.J. (1974) 'The Nurse as a Behavioural Engineer', *Nursing Times*, 70, pp. 1396-7

Cockrill, V.K. and Bernal, M.E. (1968) 'Operant Conditioning of Verbal Behaviour in a Withdrawn Patient by a Patient Peer', *Perspectives in Psychiatric Care*, 6, pp. 230-7

Comley, R. (1976) 'Self-injurious Behaviour in a Retarded Child', *Nursing Mirror*, 142, pp. 66-7

Docherty, P. (1978) 'Success is Sweet as John Speaks Up', *Nursing Mirror*, 147, pp.45-7

Eveleigh, C. (1977) 'Behavioural Psychotherapy to Encourage Self-treatment of a Patient with Obsessive–Compulsive Neurosis', *Nursing Times*, 73, pp.1036-8

Farrington, A. (1983) 'Obsessive–Compulsive Disorder', *Nursing Mirror*, 157, pp.326-7

193

Gelfand, D.M., Gelfand, S. and Dobson, W.R. (1967) 'Unprogrammed Reinforcement of Patients' Behaviour in a Mental Hospital', *Behaviour Research and Therapy*, 5, pp. 201-7

Gilbert, M.T. (1976) 'A Behavioural Approach to Child Abuse', *Nursing Times*, 72, pp. 140-3

Goldberg, D.P., Bridges, K., Cooper, W., Hyde, C., Sterling, C. and Wyatt, R. (1985) 'Douglas House: A New Type of Hostel Ward for Chronic Psychotic Patients', *British Journal of Psychiatry*, 147, pp. 383-8

Gray, M. (1972) 'Behaviour Modification in a Long-term Psychiatric Ward', *Nursing Times*, 68, pp.540-1

Hardin, S.B. and Durham, J.D. (1985) 'Exploring the Structure, Process and Effectiveness of Nurse Psychotherapists', *Psychosocial Nursing and Mental Health Services*, 23, pp. 8-15

Hartie, A. and Black, D. (1975) 'A Dry Bed is the Objective', *Nursing Times*, 71, pp. 1874-6

Hersen, M. and Barlow, D.H. (1976) *Single Case Experimental Designs: Strategies for Studying Behavior Change*, Pergamon, New York

Joyce, J. and Dustin, G. (1982) 'Active Analysis', *Nursing Mirror*, 155, pp. 14-16

Linke, S. (1982) 'Behaviour Analysis in the Care of the Elderly', *Nursing Times*, 78, pp.656-8

Manchester, J. (1981) 'Child Abuse and its Prevention: A Behavioural Approach', *Nursing Times*, 77, pp.478-90

Marks, I.M. (1973) 'The Psychiatric Nurse as a Therapist: Developments and Problems', *Nursing Times*, 69, pp. 137-9

Marks, I.M., Hallam, R.S., Connolly, J. and Philpott, R. (1977) *Nursing in Behavioural Psychotherapy*, Royal College of Nursing, London

Mercer, S. (1984) 'Obsessive Compulsive Disorder', *Nursing Times*, 157, pp. 33-7

Merchant, J. and Saxby, P. (1981) 'Reality Orientation: A Way Forward', *Nursing Times*, 77, pp. 1442-4

Milne, D. (1984) 'The Development and Evaluation of a Structured Learning Format Introduction to Behaviour Therapy for Psychiatric Nurses', *British Journal of Clinical Psychology*, 23, pp. 175-85

Milne, D. (1986) *Training Behaviour Therapists: Methods, Evaluation and Implementation with Parents, Nurses and Teachers*, Croom Helm, London/Brookline Books, Cambridge, Mass.

Milne, D., Burdett, C. and Conway, P. (1985) 'Review and Replication of a 'Core Course' in Behaviour Therapy for Psychiatric Nurses', *Journal of Advanced Nursing*, 10, pp.137-48

Moore, P. and Carr, J. (1976) 'Behaviour Modification Programme', *Nursing Times*, 72, pp. 1356-7

Morrice, J.K.W. (1980) Correspondence, *British Journal of Psychiatry*, 136, pp. 106-7

O'Brien, P., Caldwell, G. and Transeau, G. (1985) 'Destroyers: Written Treatment Contracts Can Help Cure Self-destructive Behaviours of Borderline Patients', *Psychosocial Nursing and Mental Health Services*, 23, pp. 19-23

Orton, D. (1979) 'Behavioural Treatment of Hyperactivity in a Mentally Handicapped Child', *Nursing Times*, 75, pp. 758-60

Patrick, A. and Rafferty, J. (1978) 'Modifying Behaviour in an Institution', *Nursing Times*, 74, pp. 1840-5

Peterson, R.F. and Peterson, L.R. (1968) 'The Use of Reinforcement in the Control of Self-destructive Behaviour in a Retarded Boy', *Journal of Experimental and Child Psychology*, 6, pp. 351-60

Pickstock, J. and Taylor, J. (1976) 'Behaviour Modification in a Severely Subnormal Child', *Nursing Mirror*, 142, pp. 216-19

Pope, C. and Buck, R. (1982) 'Spoonful of Success', *Nursing Mirror*, 155, pp. 14-16

Prehn, R.A. (1982) 'Applied Behaviour Analysis for Disturbed Elderly Patients', *Journal of Gerontological Nursing*, 8 May, pp. 286-8

Reavley, W. and Herdman, L.F. (1985) 'Training Nurses in Behavioural Psychotherapy', *British Journal of Medical Psychology*, 58, pp. 249-56

Savage, S. and Biley, F. (1984) 'Bulimia Nervosa', *Nursing Times*, 80, pp.42-5

Sawyer, N. (1983) 'A Fear of Cancer', *Nursing Mirror*, 17 Aug. (Mental Health Forum), pp. iii–vii

Schmidt, M.P.W. and Duncan, B.A.B. (1974) 'Modifying Eating Behavior in Anorexia Nervosa', *American Journal of Nursing*, 74, pp. 1646-8

Scottish National Nursing and Midwifery Consultative Committee (1976) 'A New Concept of Nursing', *Nursing Times* (Occasional paper), 72, pp. 49-52

Seidel, H. and Hodgkinson, P. (1979) 'Behaviour Modification and Long-term Learning in Korsakoff's Psychosis', *Nursing Times*, 75, pp. 1855-7

Sewpaul, C., Thorpe, J.G. and Tyerman, C. (1982) 'Control of Body-rocking in a Mentally Handicapped Boy', *Nursing Times*, 78, pp. 1045-7

Simpson, S.D. (1982) 'Treatment of Sexual Dysfunction by Behavioural Psychotherapy', *Nursing Times*, 78, pp. 57-8

Slater, V. (1982) 'A Behavioural Programme for Billy', *Nursing Times*, 78, pp. 1267-8

Smith, A. (1984) 'The Token Economy: Does it Work?' *Nursing Times*, 80, pp. 64-5

Tamez, E.G., Moore, M.J. and Brown, P.L. (1978) 'Relaxation Training as a Nursing Intervention Versus PRN Medication', *Nursing Research*, 27, pp. 160-5

Tilley, S. (1985) 'Multiple Phobias and Grief: a Case Study', *Behavioural Psychotherapy*, 13, pp. 59-68

Ward, M.F. (1985) *The Nursing Process in Psychiatry*, Churchill Livingstone, Edinburgh

Williamson, F. (1974) 'The Fourth is Freedom from Fear', *Nursing Times*, 70, pp. 1840-2

Woods, P.A. and Cullen, C. (1983) 'Determinants of Staff Behaviour in Long-term Care', *Behavioural Psychotherapy*, 11, pp. 4-17

10

Evaluation in Occupational Therapy

Margaret Nicol

EDITOR'S INTRODUCTION

Although occupational therapy is a relatively young profession, there is already an awareness of the need to base future developments on careful evaluation. This is reflected in the increased prominence accorded to research methods in occupational therapists' (OTs) education. Margaret Nicol summarises the main methods that have been used by OTs, namely case studies, surveys, correlational studies and quasi-experimental research designs. She concludes that this emphasis on research can help OTs to justify their treatment methods, determine the relative efficacy of alternative treatments, and generally promote professional success and independence.

10.1 INTRODUCTION

Occupational therapy is a developing profession only now coming out of its infancy. It has, like many other developing professions, concerned itself with establishing an identity, evolving treatment regimes and educating future occupational therapists (OTs). It has tended to 'borrow' theories and knowledge from areas such as medicine and psychology and fit them into an occupational therapy framework. Evaluation of these treatment regimes has been neglected as OTs tend to see themselves primarily as clinicians and not researchers.

As we move into the 1990s, OTs and their consumers are

beginning to be more concerned about the effectiveness of treatment. The occupational therapy profession is beginning to develop a more research-orientated approach as it is essential that the field of occupational therapy becomes independent in developing its own theories and areas of practice. These theories and resultant practice must be evaluated in a scientific way if occupational therapy wishes to become a respected profession.

Gibson (1984) states that 'little research has been conducted and published in the area of mental health occupational therapy, despite the growth of occupational therapy in general and despite research efforts in speciality areas other than mental health.' She postulates the following reasons for this;

(1) Small numbers of occupational therapists with research degrees or the experience to supervise other occupational therapists wishing to undertake research.

(2) The problems of conducting research in mental health: the validity of studies can be questioned because of difficulties in determining homogeneous populations and because theories and treatment are difficult to define. These are problems shared by other mental health workers.

(3) The lack of a theoretical framework for occupational therapy in psychiatry. This is currently being addressed by OTs (Reilly, 1962; Kielhofner and Burke, 1980; Hemphill, 1982; Reed and Sanderson, 1983; Barris, Kielhofner and Watts, 1983). Progress is slowly being achieved.

(4) The level of research taught in occupational therapy education: occupational therapy tends to attract and educate people who want to be clinicians. It does not place a great emphasis on research. However, this is changing and increasingly courses are including more research in the curriculum.

(5) Occupational therapy is predominantly a female profession and many experienced researchers leave the profession because of family commitments, diminishing the pool of experienced people available to supervise junior members of the profession in their research efforts.

10.2 RESEARCH METHODS

In acknowledging the limitations of research in occupational therapy it is important to recognise the importance of that which has been done. Occupational therapists have tended to use the following research designs:

(a) The case study

This is a descriptive research design consisting of an in-depth study of a single subject. The research material is collected over a period of time in a 'natural' or clinical setting, as opposed to a laboratory environment. There are advantages and disadvantages to this type of study (see Cox and West, 1983, for further discussion on this). Davis (1985) used this approach to illustrate the role of occupational therapy in child psychiatry. She described the case of Anne, who was referred because of sexual abuse. There is a brief outline of Anne's social history followed by more extensive detail on the occupational therapy treatment sessions, mainly involving the use of painting. In the short discussion Davis concludes that by using the case study she 'highlights how the occupational therapist with her focus on the individual can make a very important contribution to the treatment of a distressed family'. This is a very descriptive study and provides further insights into sexual abuse. It may also be useful in further investigations exploring child sexual abuse, and in particular the use of painting as a way of exploring the child's emotions. Leveille (1981) used a similar approach, the sensory integrative approach (SIA) to explore the use of the sensory integrative SIA with a chronic, tactile, defensive schizophrenic. In describing the case of Richard, Leveille outlines his difficulties and his abilities before commencing techniques using an SIA. These techniques involve activities which will provide kinaesthetic and vestibular stimulation and attempt to reintegrate the vestibular system which is thought to be disorganised in chronic schizophrenia. In comparing Richard's difficulties and abilities following treatment improvements are identified, and these are maintained after a period of time. Care must be used in interpreting data from single-subject studies and Leveille suggests that 'this experiment indicates that sensory integration needs still further exploration'. She hoped that this study would stimulate OTs to pursue sensory integrative techniques.

(b) The survey

This research design is used when gathering information from a group of people. It is still a descriptive study but is cross-sectional and the material is collected from a group of individuals at one point in time. The data collected relate to what is happening rather than why this is so. The survey should be designed to get answers to specific questions. Occupational therapists have used this method to obtain information concerning clients/patients or to obtain information from fellow OTs/other professionals. Anderson, (1985), for instance, undertook a survey to determine the degree to which OTs working in mental health settings were assessing the work potential of patients. She surveyed 500 therapists and received 231 replies, of which 157 were used as part of the study. A questionnaire consisting of 20 items required the respondents to indicate the usage of standardised and non-standardised tests. Work has been a part of the basis for treatment throughout the history of the occupational therapy profession, but despite this historical emphasis only 56 OTs sampled (36 per cent) were actually evaluating work potential. The remaining 101 saw the need for this type of evaluation and would like to incorporate it into their programmes. In the survey done by Anderson 75 per cent of the 56 occupational therapists undertaking work performance evaluation used crafts as their assessment tool. Sixty-five per cent used non-standardised measures, and only 23 per cent used standardised tests. Anderson recommends that there is a need for more information about work performance evaluations and about the type of patients appropriate for them. Occupational therapists need to become more aware that their observations of patient work potential must be accurate and more of these observations need to be substantiated by the use of objective data.

Jeffrey, Lyne and Redfern (1984) undertook a survey among OTs to establish the extent of occupational therapy services in the field of child and adolescent psychiatry within the National Health Service in Britain. Questionnaires were sent to all health authorities in Britain asking them to identify child and adolescent services with an input from occupational therapy. Further questionnaires were then sent to identified units. Data were obtained on staffing structures, facilities, post-registration training and research activities. They showed that child and adolescent psychiatry is a popular field of work for OTs and that there is a need for further post-registration training. This has implications for health authorities, the College of Occupational Therapists and the OTs in this field of practice to provide appropriate courses to meet this need.

(c) Experimental and quasi-experimental studies

These are often considered to be 'true' research. They concern themselves with why things happen, i.e. the cause-and-effect relationship between independent and dependent variables. For example, treatments can be compared to establish effective elements. Ottenbacher and Short (1982) surveyed articles appearing in the *American Journal of Occupational Therapy* over the past decade. They concluded that there has been a significant change in the type of articles published before and after 1978. There has been an increase in articles of a quasi-experimental nature and a decrease in articles of a purely descriptive type. It would seem that OTs are moving towards more scientific methods of enquiry.

De Carlo and Mann (1985) studied the effectiveness of verbal versus activity groups in improving self-perceptions of interpersonal communication skills. Their design was of a pre-test, post-test and control group type. Subjects were defined and then randomly allocated to one of three groups: (a) an experimental group that received activity therapy, (b) an experimental group that received verbal therapy, (c) a control group that was involved in the normal work of the centre but did not specifically participate in activities aimed at improving communication skills. The groups were assessed and those receiving specific treatment met for 8 weeks and all groups were then reassessed. A description of the various treatment sessions was given. The authors concluded from their data that the group that was involved in activity therapy attained a significantly higher level of interpersonal communication skills than the group that was involved in verbal therapy. However, neither the activity group nor the verbal group performed significantly better than the control group. The authors then discussed the limitations of the study. They point out that the value of verbal groups is well accepted by mental health workers but that the value of activity groups is less well understood. The findings of the study suggest that further research into activity groups would be valuable. This may influence other mental health workers' views and knowledge on the use of activity groups.

Campbell and McCreadie (1983) used a similar method to determine whether occupational therapy was effective for chronic schizophrenic day patients. Having defined their patient population they identified one experimental group and one control group. Each patient was assessed and then randomly allocated to the two groups. Treatment was carried out for 12 weeks followed by reassessment. The results indicated improvement, particularly in laundry and household skills. The authors in reporting these results do not indicate if these are statistically significant. A follow-up study was proposed in order to see if these improvements were maintained. They do point out that these improved skills are the important ones to help the person function more successfully in the community.

(d) Correlational studies

This type of research design is used to determine the degree of relationship between two or more variables. Gregory (1983) conducted a survey to study the correlation between occupational behaviour and life satisfaction among retirees. He reviewed the literature and concluded that studies are needed to determine the meaning of activities in retirement that substitute for work, to see whether the satisfaction derived from worker roles continues in the activities of retirement. He surveyed subjects chosen from a variety of settings for the elderly in Richmond, Virginia. Seventy-nine people successfully completed the questionnaire he had designed. Gregory found a significant correlation between life satisfaction and occupational behaviour. He suggested that this correlation had clinical implications and that OTs should be evaluating what function the activity serves for the retired persons, not just what activities they are engaged in. This may be important in promoting healthy lifestyles among elderly people.

10.3 CONCLUSION

Occupational therapists must become more aware that their

treatment methods have to be justified. Research can help OTs to answer important questions about which of their treatment methods are most effective. In doing this it will help promote the success of the occupational therapy profession, foster professional independence and help acquire an equal status with other professions. Occupational therapists are becoming involved in research.

REFERENCES

Anderson, A.P. (1985) 'Work Potential Evaluation in Mental Health, *American Journal of Occupational Therapy, 39*, pp. 659-63

Barris, R., Keilhofner, G. and Watts, J.H. (1983) *Psychosocial Occupational Therapy*, Ramsco Publishing, Laurel, Maryland

Campbell, A. and McCreadie, R.G. (1983) 'Occupational Therapy is Effective for Chronic Schizophrenic Day Patients', *British Journal of Occupational Therapy, 46*, pp. 327-9

Cox, R.C. and West, W.L. (1983) *Fundamentals of Research for Health Professionals*, Ramsco Publishing, Laurel, Maryland

Davis, S. (1985) 'The Role of the Occupational Therapists in Child Psychiatry: a Case Illustration,' *British Journal of Occupational Therapy, 48*, pp. 266-8

DeCarlo, J.J. and Mann, W.C. (1985) 'The Effectiveness of Verbal Versus Activity Groups in Improving Self-Perceptions of Interpersonal Communication Skills', *American Journal of Occupational Therapy, 39*, pp. 20-7

Gibson, B. (1984) 'The Dearth of Mental Health Research in Occupational Therapy', *Occupational Therapy Journal of Research, 4*, pp. 131-50

Gregory, M.D. (1983) 'Occupational Behaviour and Life Satisfaction Among Retirees', *American Journal of Occupational Therapy, 37*, pp. 548-60

Hemphill, B. (1982) *The Evaluative Process on Psychiatric Occupational Therapy*, Charles Slack Inc., Thorofare, N.J.

Kielhofner, G. and Burke, J.P. (1980) 'A Model of Human Occupation', *American Journal of Occupational Therapy, 34*, pp. 573-81

Leveille, J. (1981) 'Outline of a Sensory Integrative Approach with a Chronic Schizophrenic', *British Journal of Occupational Therapy, 44*, pp. 160-3

Ottenbacher, K. and Short, M.A. (1982) 'Publication Trends in Occupational Therapy', *Occupational Therapy Journal of Research, 2*, pp. 80-9

Reed, K. and Sanderson, S. (1983) *Concepts of Occupational Therapy*, Williams & Wilkins, Baltimore

Reilly, M. (1962) 'Occupational Therapy Can Be One of the Great Ideas of the Twentieth Century', *American Journal of Occupational Therapy, 16*, pp. 1-9

11

Evaluation in Psychiatry:
Planning, Developing and Evaluating
Community-based Mental Health Services for Adults

Ian Falloon, Greg Wilkinson, Judith Burgess and Sheila
McLees

EDITOR'S INTRODUCTION

Falloon and his colleagues begin by presenting a systems
model that is relevant to their concern to meet patient needs
in an efficient way. This model concentrates on needs assessment, goal-setting, resource allocation, action, progress
reviews and outcome statements. Each of these elements is
discussed in terms of planning a relevant and systematic
approach to community care, harnessing informal and formal
resources. The difficulties in arranging for a truly experimental analysis of this model are acknowledged and epidemiological methods are suggested as a practical alternative.
Cost-efficiency is also emphasised. This approach, elaborated
in a review of relevant research work, suggests that a
community-based, 24-hour care service would prove more
effective than the traditional hospital-based approach in
reducing the prevalence of chronic mental disorders and
associated social handicaps.

This is a cogent and powerful case for community care,
linked to the introduction of coherent models and objectively
verified treatment programmes. Few stones are left unturned
and many mental health practitioners will find encouragement in the purposeful blend of empiricism and pragmatism
that this chapter exemplifies.

11.1 INTRODUCTION

The use of the term 'community' to describe recent changes in the provision of mental health services would imply that earlier services were not oriented towards the needs of the communities in which they were based. This was certainly true of the Victorian mental asylums, built in rural settings at some distance from the urban communities from whence most of their inmates came and few returned. The rehousing of the chronically mentally ill and resiting of hospital wards for the acutely mentally ill in urban areas, often within general hospital complexes, may reduce the physical distance between the service and the community served, but it does not always reduce the psychological distance between the community and the service. Indeed, it may well increase the negative attitudes towards the services, unless relocation is associated with significant reductions in the unmet mental health needs of the community. Thus, planning a new community psychiatric service requires much greater consideration than mere relocation of patients, staff and resources.

(a) An evaluative model for the development and evaluation of a community psychiatric service

A successful service to a community is one that meets all the relevant needs with maximum efficiency and minimal costs (economic *and* emotional).

The model proposed by John Raeburn (Raeburn and Seymour, 1977) in Auckland, New Zealand, provides an excellent example of a systematic approach to planning this process (Figure 11.1). The initial step involves the accurate assessment of the current needs of the defined population. The more precisely these needs can be defined in terms of types of psychiatric disorders, frequencies of sufferers and the severity, the more accurately the appropriate resources required to reduce this morbidity can be estimated. Before the resource allocation step it is crucial that the goals of the service are clearly defined. The goals need to be realistic, clearly operationalised and readily assessed. Clearly, conditions for which no current effective treatment is available may necessitate quite different goals to preventable, curable disorders. Resource allocation must be targeted towards the task of achieving the goals. Where resources are clearly insufficient to provide effective interventions to achieve all the goals, priorities may need to be set

Figure 11.1: Basic systems model (only two of several possible feedback loops are shown)

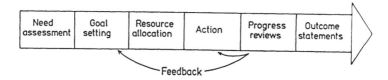

and more limited goals targeted. The implementation step involves application of the most cost-effective technology to the task of achieving the goals of the service. This often includes the training of staff in the technical skills required, as well as considering the settings under which the application of these skills is most effective and efficient. Regular and continuous review of the effectiveness of the methods employed is an essential part of the feedback process, which enables efficient adjustment to strategy where necessary. Less frequent major reviews of the achievement of the goals and the changing pattern of needs for the service forms the final step. The continuous evaluation and constructive feedback achieved through this model enables the service to respond rapidly to the changing needs of the community, changes in the allocation and provision of resources and to refinements in the technical skills implemented.

(b) Defining community needs

The most crucial step in establishing a community service is pinpointing the needs of that community. Ideally, this would involve an extensive survey of all persons in the community to ascertain the exact prevalence and incidence of all forms of mental disorder. Such surveys are impossible in clinical practice. Usually planners resort to counting cases currently receiving specialised management (outpatient, day patient, inpatient), occasionally with special assistance of community case registers (Gibbons, Jennings and Wing, 1981). However, as Goldberg and Huxley (1980) have pointed out, such procedures provide a very inadequate measure of the actual prevalence of mental illness in a community, and grossly underestimate the needs of that community.

Fortunately, a number of excellent community-based surveys of the prevalence of mental disorders have been conducted in recent years that provide an excellent guide to the likely needs of a community in terms of management of established disorders. The use of standardised diagnostic schedules and sophisticated epidemiological methods (Regier, Burke, Manderscheid and Burns, 1985) enables us to generalise the findings of these studies to some extent. The two most comprehensive surveys — one in rural Bavaria (Dilling and Weyrerer, 1984), the other in five divergent urban centres in the United States (Regier, Myers, Kramer *et al.*, 1984), suggest, at least in industrialised cultures, that the prevalence of the major mental disorders is strikingly similar. Although there is evidence that in non-industrialised societies the patterns of prevalence of mental disorders may differ substantially from those found in the industrialised world (WHO, in preparation), it seems reasonable to plan community services in Britain on the basis of these epidemiological data.

Despite the absence of major epidemiological research on the prevalence of mental disorders in Britain, studies of mental health consultation patterns to the well-developed primary care services provide a reasonable estimate of the prevalence of known needs of the community (Goldberg and Huxley, 1980; Shepherd, Cooper, Brown and Kalton, 1966). However, these figures do not include a substantial proportion of the mentally disordered who do not consult with their general practitioners. Surprisingly, this population includes many cases of quite severe impairment and associated handicap. Thus the identification of all cases who would benefit from mental health management and the provision of services that facilitate management of such cases by the appropriate resources is a crucial goal for an effective service to the community.

The two most striking features derived from the prevalence data are first, that one-fifth of the population will suffer a definable mental disorder in the course of one year, i.e. 200 in every 1000; of whom 30–50 per 1000 are deemed severe cases requiring specialist services, and three to five at any time requiring 24-hour care services. Secondly, such extensive community needs far exceed the current capacity of hospital-based service provision. A minimum of 300 hospital places would be required for a population of 100,000 and 3,000 cases would need to be provided with outpatient services each year. Furthermore, it is of interest to note that although our current models of hospital-based services are set up primarily to manage the functional psychoses (mainly schizophrenia and manic-depressive psychosis), these conditions have a low prevalence in the community. Thus, it seems likely that our current allocation of resources does not reflect the actual needs of the community and may be a major factor in the dissatisfaction expressed about psychiatric institutions and the resulting political pressure for change.

(c) Definition of the goals of mental health services

The goals of most mental health services are poorly defined. The usual goal would appear to be to meet the needs of all cases referred to the service. Such lack of specificity leads to inevitable failure. Referral agents tend to seek specialist consultation for a variety of reasons, many of which have little relevance to the service. Requests for patients to be admitted to mental hospitals tend to relate as much to the social needs of the community caregivers as to the need for intensive medical assessment and treatment (Wing, 1968; Parkes, 1978). Psychiatric hospitals have long provided a respite or asylum from the social stresses of the community, and as a result have become an important provider of 24-hour *social* care and emergency housing. Medical labels are readily accorded to troubled persons who appear 'anxious', 'depressed', 'hopeless', 'suicidal' and 'distraught'. Indeed, even with the revised Mental Health Act (1983) non-medical disorders such as psychopathy are included in the classification of mental disorders, and social needs appear to take precedence over medical needs. In a survey of hospital admissions in North Buckinghamshire only one in every nine cases was admitted specifically for medical treatment (Burgess, personal communication).

It would seem crucial that the goals of a mental health service must be tailored to the specific needs of the mentally ill persons in the community. This must include efforts to prevent mental illness, in particular those severe disorders that tend to become chronic. Such efforts would seek to achieve the ultimate goal of reducing the *prevalence* of mental illness in that community. Secondary goals would include the detection of persons with a high risk of mental illness and primary prevention efforts; the detection of early signs of mental illness and secondary prevention efforts (through effective early treatment); the provision of effective treatment of established mental illness to prevent chronicity and secondary handicaps; and the provision of effective rehabilitation of persons with existing chronic disorders and associated handicaps.

The provision of social care and psychosocial counselling for persons with psychological problems that are not associated with current or impending mental illness must be viewed as a secondary activity, that can only be considered when clear evidence of a reducing prevalence of mental illness is achieved. Problems such as family and marital discord, social inadequacy, violence, anti-social behaviour and the responses to life stresses should be considered to fall within the ambit of the mental health service only when they are associated with a mental illness or there is clearly a *high* risk of the development of a chronic mental illness. However, it may be important that such persons receive adequate assessment and are screened for the presence or high risk of mental illness. Thus, consultation and support for the development of effective management of such persons within social and psychological services is an important goal of the mental health service.

(d) Organisation and allocation of resources

It seems of vital importance that the resources available within a community are sufficient to meet the goals of the service, and as a result, the needs of that community. The absence of careful planning, or planning based upon the *laissez-faire* goals of providing a service based upon referrals to outpatient clinics or admissions to hospital, has led to a situation where the resources allocated by the health services bear little relationship to the *actual* needs of the community. Health service planning continues to be based upon the number of 'hospital beds' required for a given population. Such concepts tend to reduce the flexibility to tailor resources to the goals and needs of the mentally ill in a community.

However, although the goal of a mental health service may involve effective management of mental illness, this does not mean that management of *all* such cases is the prerogative of the specialist service alone. In the UK it is estimated that between 90 and 95 per cent of all cases of mental illness are managed by the primary care services (mainly general practitioners) (Goldberg and Huxley, 1980; Shepherd et al., 1966). This percentage is somewhat lower in Europe (Dilling and Weyrerer, 1984) and the US (Regier et al., 1985). In the UK mental illness remains one of the few areas of medicine where the techological revolution has not usurped the role of the GP as case manager. Few GPs are eager to have this aspect of patient care removed entirely from their jurisdiction, and most state their clear preference that they continue their case management role but welcome the consultation of a specialist mental health service to support their case management.

Community resources extend beyond general practitioners. The health visitors and other community nurses who comprise the primary care service all provide a substantial amount of care to the mentally ill. Health visitors are expected to provide a major role in the prevention of illness and in health promotion. Their work is ideally suited to assist in the prevention and early detection of mental illness, particularly disorders found in young families and the elderly. Once again, they prefer to enhance this role with the consultation and support of mental health professionals rather than merely handing over cases to the specialist service.

Perhaps the most undervalued resources for the management of mental illness in the community are the patients' families and close associates. Hospital-based services have shown little acknowledgement of the vital role families play in the care of the mentally ill. At best their efforts have been taken for granted, at worst they have been accused of playing a major role in the aetiology of mental illness. However, unquestionably the family is the greatest community resource for the management of mental illness. With a modicum of respect and support the caregiving efforts of families can be readily extended to provide excellent care for their mentally ill members. Furthermore, by dint of their experience as caregivers many family members have acquired skills in the management of severe disorders which may assist the professional services. Thus, consultation must always be viewed as a two-way process. As well as providing an advisory role some skilled family members may play a more direct role in the development of mental health services as volunteers, foster parents and in leading family support groups.

Finally, existing community resources include a wide range of non-medical services that provide a substantial amount of care and support for the mentally ill. These include specific voluntary organisations such as the National Association of Mental Health (MIND), the National Schizophrenia Fellowship, or Alcoholics Anonymous. However, social agencies such as the local authority social services, police, Citizens' Advice Bureaux, as well as the churches and other community-oriented bodies, also provide a substantial resource for mental health care.

The widely disparate and informal nature of many of these resources suggests the need for a well co-ordinated mental health policy that effectively harnesses and provides clear direction for the non-specialised efforts. Before developing alternative services it is important that these resources are carefully evaluated in terms of the precise services they provide and the major community needs that cannot be met through cost-effective training and support for their activities. Thus, the establishment of a mental health service to a community should seek to complement existing services rather than supplant them. The vast numbers of cases of mental illness that exist in a community can never be handled entirely by a specialised service. It is important that the specialist service provides guidance, consultation and co-ordination for the informal services, assisting them to improve the efficiency of their work. To date no service has been developed along these lines, although Shepherd and his colleagues (1966) advocated such a development two decades ago. Until now, services to a community have been developed with the hospital as the base with the vast majority of resources concentrated on the 24-hour care of less than 1 per cent of the mentally ill in that community. The questions have not been asked, at least not in the UK, as to whether this is the most efficient use of specialist resources, and whether the community needs are effectively met by these hospital-based resources. This is a matter that requires urgent evaluation.

A final important consideration concerns the quality of the professional skills of the specialist personnel allocated to the mental health service. Because the training of most mental health professionals is largely oriented to hospital-based practice, there is a substantial discrepancy between their skills and the community needs. Anxiety disorders, minor depression and uncomplicated schizophrenia are conditions seldom seen in hospital-based practice; nor are the psychosocial aspects of long-term community management, such as the work with families, GPs, health visitors and social services part of the basic training. A lack of technical skills in these areas may seriously restrict the mental health professional in community-based work. For this reason a substantial training effort is essential for all staff at all levels. This should focus on training in procedures that have demonstrated cost-effectiveness with the target needs to which they will be applied. The evaluation of efficient training programmes is another crucial area for urgent attention (Milne, 1986).

(e) Implementing the programme and evaluating progress and outcome

The implementation of a mental health service will depend upon the effectiveness of the planning stages, including the recruitment and technical training of personnel. The provision of good administrative procedures that ensure the efficient operation of the programme is crucial. This includes procedures that enable monitoring the effectiveness of all aspects of the service. Regular review allows the early detection of emerging problems and their resolution before major crises develop. It also permits positive feedback for progress.

Whereas factorial designs with random assignment and blind assessment are seldom feasible for service evaluation, epidemiological methods may provide an alternative approach. If the needs of the community are being met the prevalence of morbidity associated with mental illness will be expected to decline. The patterns of this decline would be expected to follow the specific needs that are targeted as major goals for the service. An economic analysis of the efficiency of services is an important consideration. The lower the cost, in terms of total community resources (including 'emotional' costs) to achieve a service goal, the more resources can be extended to other goals. For example, if a health visitor can treat a case of postnatal depression, with GP assistance, as effectively as a psychologist and psychiatrist, and at a lower cost, the former management should be advocated. The same primary care resource may find management of a severe case of puerperal psychosis beyond their skills, and the specialist team may prove more efficient case managers. Such decisions can be made readily in a well-organised community-based service where skills can be applied in the most efficient manner to resolve problems on a case-by-case basis.

The next section of this chapter will provide a selective review of the various components of a mental health service in an attempt to define the extent of knowledge of the effectiveness of community-based approaches to mental health care.

11.2 SPECIALIST LIAISON WITH THE GENERAL PRACTITIONER

In contrast to the large volume of work relating to minor psychiatric morbidity in primary care, very little attention has been paid to serious mental disorders in this setting (Wilkinson, 1985; Wilkinson and Freeman, 1986; Shepherd et al., 1986). Shepherd et al. (1966) found that about 14 per cent of general practice patients consulted their doctor at least once in a 12-month period for a condition diagnosed as largely, or entirely, psychiatric in nature. Just over half of these patients had chronic conditions, defined as those continuously present for at least 1 year, or recurring with sufficient frequency to cause continuous disability or to require continuous prophylactic treatment. These findings have generally been confirmed by subsequent workers. In an important US study (Regier et al., 1985) about 30 per cent of primary care patients were found to have a diagnosis of mental disorder, and five-sixths of these disorders had a duration of over 1 year. Both studies are in agreement that about 8 per cent of patients seen in a primary care setting suffer from chronic mental disorders with some degree of functional impairment. Within this heterogeneous group of disorders, affective disorders have the highest overall rates of occurrence, but psychotic, anxiety and personality disorders contribute the greatest proportion of severe disability.

(a) The role of the general practitioner in the care of the chronically mentally ill

Much of the burden of medical care for patients with mental disorders falls, inevitably, on the general practitioner. This is illustrated by the pattern of care that emerged from a survey of chronically mentally ill patients in North Buckinghamshire (see Figure 11.2). In the course of 1 year, patients consulted general practitioners more than twice as frequently as they consulted mental health services; and general practitioners had three times the number of emergency consultations as did the mental health services. Over a quarter of all the patients' consultations were for non-psychiatric complaints. The bulk of specialised mental health services were provided by community psychiatric nurses (CPNs). Care by the psychiatrist was limited to less than 10 per cent of the overall patient contacts with medical services. These findings fit in well with the observation by Shepherd *et al.* (1966) that the great bulk of identified cases of mental disorder are dealt with by the practitioners themselves. At the same time, it should not be forgotten that perhaps a quarter of those patients suffering from chronic mental disorders may not come to the attention of either general practitioners or psychiatrists (Johnstone, Owens, Gold *et al.*, 1984).

Figure 11.2: Care of the chronically mentally ill by North Buckinghamshire general practitioners and the Buckingham mental health service, April 1984–April 1985

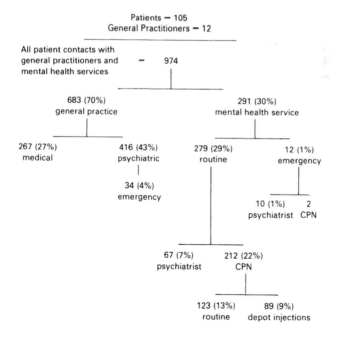

(b) Options for improving the management of patients with mental disorders in general practice

There are disappointingly few empirical clinical studies *from general practice* upon which firm recommendations about improvements in management, including drug management, might be based. Drugs apart, however, three crucial elements stand out: psychiatrist/general practitioner liaison–consultation attachment schemes; the therapeutic role of community nurses and social workers; and the family-based management of psychiatric disorders.

Unfortunately, few psychiatrist/general practitioner liaison–consultation attachment schemes have been evaluated (Strathdee and Williams, 1984). In Tyrer's (1984) experience, the patients seen in general practice psychiatric clinics encompass the entire range of psychiatric disorders. A significant proportion have chronic mental disorders, and almost half are still attending the clinic at the end of a 2-year period. Most patients are treated in the clinic, sometimes seeing the community nurse, or by other members of the primary care team, including health visitors and district nurses. Patients apparently prefer such clinics to hospital clinics because of the ease of access and the relative absence of stigma. When Tyrer, Seivewright and Wollerton (1984) compared the frequency of contacts with the psychiatric services for patients from practices with and without such psychiatric clinics, the effects of the clinics appeared to be: most importantly, a 20 per cent fall in the number of admissions to psychiatric hospital; an increase in the number of outpatients seen; and a fall in the number of new referrals. The clinics were also associated with a relative increase in the number of domiciliary visits and an increase in acute day hospital referrals.

Two randomised controlled clinical trials have shown clinical and economic benefits in favour of community nursing for neurotic patients. In one study (Paykel, Mangen, Griffith and Burns, 1982) neurotic patients requiring follow-up (mean total life-time psychiatric treatment received about 40 months) were assigned to routine psychiatric outpatient care or to supportive home visiting from community psychiatric nurses. No differences were found between the effectiveness of the two modes of service on symptoms, social adjustment or family burden, at up to 18 months follow-up. Community psychiatric nursing resulted in a marked reduction in outpatient contacts with psychiatrists and other staff, more discharges, and a small increase in general practitioner contact for prescribing. In the other investigation (Marks, 1985), neurotic patients with mainly phobic and obsessive–compulsive disorders (mean duration 7 years) did better up to 1 year follow-up after receiving behavioural psychotherapy from a nurse therapist rather than routine treatment from a general practitioner. As before, in both cases patients preferred being treated in the primary care setting.

In a recent controlled trial of the effectiveness of social work for depressed women in general practice (Corney, 1984), women suffering from acute or acute-on-chronic depression were randomly allocated to routine treatment by their doctor or referral to an attached social worker. Sixty per cent of both groups were clinically improved at 6-month follow-up. However, women assessed initially as suffering from acute-on-chronic depression with major marital difficulties were found to benefit from social work intervention. These patients could be distinguished from the others by their high degree of motivation, the initial severity of their problems and by the amount of practical help provided by the social workers.

It is concluded that there is no established, empirically based, comprehensive and integrated approach to the psychopharmacological, social and psychological treatment of patients with mental disorders in primary care. The questions of how to determine what balance of physical, social and psychological care is appropriate in local circumstances for specific patients, and who should give appropriate care, are still largely unanswered. Care, in this context, is also likely to mean including attention to patients' occupational, educational and domestic functioning. Primary care physicians, general practitioners, and hospital specialists, need to be trained not only to detect patients with chronic mental disorders, but also how to organise and provide early and continuing treatment for them, and to recognise when specialist mental health consultation and referral is likely to be helpful.

11.3 OUTPATIENT SERVICES

The question of whether outpatient services for the mentally ill are provided in a specialised clinical location in a hospital or health centre is a highly pragmatic one. However, it may be important to take a step back for a moment to examine the evidence to support the efficacy of specialist outpatient care of the major mental disorders in the first place. Is there evidence that the technical expertise of the mental health specialist applied in outpatient settings improves the long-term course of mental disorders to a greater extent than the care and support provided by non-specialised or informal caregivers in the community? Over the past two or three decades a number of adequately designed evaluative studies have provided evidence that, at least for some disorders, specific technical skills exist to manage efficiently most of the major mental disorders.

(a) Anxiety disorders

A large body of well-controlled research has provided evidence that the major anxiety disorders of agoraphobia and obsessive–compulsive disorders can be significantly improved through the careful application of behaviour therapy methods (Marks, 1981). The methods and results have been replicated repeatedly in numerous centres. While the results of behaviour therapy are somewhat less impressive when compared with other psychological treatment methods in the management of a broad range of disorders presenting at a psychiatric outpatient clinic (Sloane, Staples, Cristol et al., 1975), there appears little dispute that they represent a major advance in the treatment of anxiety. Serious limitations remain in the treatment of obsessive–compulsive disorders where ruminative thinking predominates. As noted earlier, the relatively straightforward nature of these methods enables less sophisticated therapists to learn to apply them in a highly effective manner.

The role of drug therapy in the management of anxiety disorders appears increasingly limited. Continuing problems of dependence and emerging evidence of harmful side-effects, particularly associated with withdrawal reactions, suggests that long-term treatment is a hazardous procedure. There seems little evidence that drugs offer any additional benefit to competent behaviour therapy for the long-term management of anxiety (Hafner and Marks, 1976; Marks, 1981), although some studies have shown that they are of equal potency in the short-term (Zitrin, Klein, Woerner and Ross, 1984).

(b) Depressive disorders

The outpatient treatment of depressive disorders is complicated by difficulties in assessment. Depressed mood is an ubiquitous feature associated with a broad range of problems, few of which can be defined as mental illnesses. Evaluative studies have adopted a wide range of definitions of depressive disorders that make comparisons hazardous.

A series of recent studies have examined the relative efficacy of antidepressant drugs and psychosocial interventions. Ten controlled studies have compared cognitive/behavioural approaches with antidepressant therapies (Beck, 1986). Five of these studies found the cognitive approaches to be more effective than antidepressant medication at the end of treatment, and not one found the psychosocial approach less efficacious than pharmacotherapy. Studies of other behavioural (Bellack, Herson and Himmelhoch, 1983) and interpersonal (Weissman, Prusoff, Dimascio et al., 1979) approaches to depression have shown similar benefits.

A major problem in evaluating the efficacy of treatment interventions in depressive disorders is that most episodes remit spontaneously over a period of a month or two. A no-treatment control is essential to compare active treatment with the natural course of the disorder. However, ethical considerations, which include the risk of suicide, preclude the use of such a control condition. Thus it is not clear whether the accepted criterion of the efficacy of antidepressant drug therapy is entirely valid, particularly when early placebo-controlled drug trials did not always support the efficacy of many of these drugs, and it is evident that the serious side-effects of these drugs reduce adherence to prescribed regimens and in some instances make the depression worse. A major collaborative study has recently been completed by the NIMH in the United States, and preliminary results offer support for the benefits of psychosocial treatment methods in mild and moderate depression with the drug therapy appearing most helpful in the more severe syndromes (Elkin, personal communication).

We have concluded that at the current state of our knowledge

217

a combination of optimal dosages of antidepressant drugs, usually tricyclic preparations, with cognitive/behavioural psychotherapeutic approaches is indicated for cases of depressive disorders. Both types of intervention are targeted to the alleviation of the specific behavioural abnormalities experienced by each case. Further research is needed to enhance the efficacy of these methods.

One additional problem is a lack of knowledge about strategies that may reduce vulnerability to recurrent episodes of depressive disorders. Social psychology studies (Vaughn and Leff, 1976; Brown and Harris, 1978) indicate that family and social stress factors may play an important role. To date no studies have demonstrated the effectiveness of psychosocial intervention in preventing recurrent depressive episodes, although one controlled study of behavioural family therapy is in progress (Follette and Jacobson, 1987). Although it has become accepted clinical practice to employ long-term antidepressant therapy in an attempt to prevent future episodes, the data are not compelling (Prien, 1984). Controlled studies suggest that the prophylactic value of continued antidepressant therapy is limited to cases where depressive features persist in a subacute fashion. Where the depressive episode remits fully no specific benefits of long-term antidepressant drugs have been detected.

There is a clear need for more controlled studies of the long-term management of depressive disorders. Clinical evidence supports efforts to reduce enduring environmental stress factors, to enhance coping with stress, including developing effective problem-solving relationships, and the judicious use of antidepressant drugs.

(c) Bipolar manic-depressive disorders

The course of bipolar disorders is characterised by recurrent episodes of severe depression or mania. Although until recently these episodes were thought to be relatively independent of environmental factors, recent research suggests that stress factors such as life events (Ambelas, 1986) and family stress (Miklowitz, Goldstein, Neuchterlein et al., in press) may increase the risk of recurrent episodes. However, to date the outpatient management has focused exclusively on reducing the frequency of episodes through drug prophylaxis. Several double-blind, placebo-controlled studies have supported the efficacy of lithium salts in enhancing the stability of patients' moods and reducing the severity of episodes (Prien, 1984). The value of long-term lithium prophylaxis has been clearly demonstrated. The limitations of this approach are less clearly defined. If careful monitoring of serum levels of lithium is maintained to sustain a non-toxic therapeutic dose range, serious side-effects remain few. But for many patients lithium prophylaxis provides only partial protection from severe episodes and the development of additional strategies is necessary. A number of drugs have shown promise, as well as psychosocial interventions aimed at reducing environmental stress factors (Falloon, Hole, Pembleton and Norris, in press). However, controlled evaluation of these innovations is lacking at present.

(d) Schizophrenia

Schizophrenia is also characterised by recurrent episodes. Although at least one-third of cases show continual symptoms, evaluative research of outpatient management has focused only on the prevention of florid symptoms. The efficacy of neuroleptic drugs in the prevention of severe exacerbations of these disorders is one of the major advances in the field of medicine this century. Davis, Schaffer, Killian et al. (1980) have summarised the numerous double-blind, placebo-controlled studies that support the outstanding effectiveness of neuroleptics in this prophylactic role. But, as with lithium in bipolar disorders, drug therapy provides only a partial answer. The yearly rate of exacerbations, although more than halved, remains around 40 per cent even when poor compliance is controlled by intra-muscular depot preparations (Hogarty, 1984).

Evidence that environmental stress may increase the risk of exacerbations has led to the addition of stress management strategies to optimal drug therapy (Falloon and Liberman, 1983). These have included studies that focus on the sufferer of schizophrenia (Hogarty, 1984; Wallace and Liberman, 1985), and more recently on the stress management potential of the patient and his/her family unit (Goldstein, Rodnick, Evans et al., 1978; Falloon, 1985; Leff, Kuipers, Berkowitz et al., 1982).

219

These studies have demonstrated consistently that the addition of psychosocial strategies aimed to enhance the long-term management of environmental stress reduces the risk of major exacerbations beyond that achieved by drug therapy alone. The most comprehensive of these studies (Falloon, 1985) compared behavioural family therapy with individual supportive psychotherapy in patients receiving optimal neuroleptic medication and community support. After 9 months the results revealed the superiority of this approach in enhancing the stability of schizophrenia, including reducing the frequency of major exacerbations as well as enhancing the rate of remission of cases with persistent symptoms. Furthermore, the clinical benefits were accompanied by enhancement of social functioning and reduced burden to the family. There was some evidence that many patients could be maintained on low doses of neuroleptics when the stress management strategy was added. These benefits continued over a 24-month period of community after-care.

Increasing concern about the serious hazards of long-term neuroleptic drug use, particularly when given in high doses, has led to a serious of studies of low-dose neuroleptic prophylaxis (Kane et al., 1983). These have included recent attempts to provide intermittent drug therapy, targeted to periods of stress where the prodromal signs of an exacerbation are recognised (Carpenter, Stephens and Rey, 1982). A controlled multi-centred collaborative study is in progress in the USA to evaluate the combined effectiveness of behavioural family therapy with standard, low-dose and targeted drug strategies on the clinical and social morbidity of schizophrenia (Schooler and Keith, 1983).

(e) Conclusions

It is apparent that specific, effective therapeutic interventions have been developed for the community management of the major mental disorders. In most cases the judicious use of drug therapy combined with broad-based psychological strategies produces the optimal results. Mental health professionals need to acquire skills in the application of these specific procedures as well as in the psychiatric and psychosocial assessment methods. Treatment methods that lack scientific validation of their effectiveness have no place in present-day mental health services. Nor, indeed, do strategies that, although effective, have been superseded by more potent or more efficient methods. Such decisions about the training in, and deployment of, appropriate technical resources must be made on purely scientific data supporting their cost-effectiveness, and should be free of ideological or philosophical considerations apart from those associated with medical ethics.

11.4 DAY TREATMENT SERVICES

There has been little co-ordination in the planning of psychiatric day hospitals and local authority day centres in the UK: they are inequitably distributed, and they vary greatly in the quality of treatment they provide (Wilkinson, 1984). Furthermore, although some form of day treatment has been available to patients with psychiatric disorders for about 40 years, little is known about the efficacy and efficiency of therapeutic practices in such settings.

(a) Methodological issues

Several evaluative studies indicate the general superiority of day hospital care over outpatient and inpatient care for patients with serious or chronic psychiatric disorders. There is, though, less consensus about the extent to which day treatment is associated with improvements in patients' symptoms, on the one hand, and, on the other, with their social adjustment. Close inspection invariably reveals that methodological inadequacies complicate the interpretation of the various investigations. For example, the number of subjects tends to be small; there may be selection bias, partial or no randomisation, or little control of such important variables as diagnosis, medication, and treatment between discharge and follow-up; day care and inpatient care are often ill-defined; outcome measures may not be standardised, nor rated blindly; and there is frequently excessive attrition of subjects during follow-up.

(b) Illustrative studies

One series of American reports (Herz, Endicott, Spitzer *et al.*,

1975; 1976, 1977; Herz, Endicott and Gibbon, 1979; Reibel and Herz, 1976; Endicott, Herz and Gibbon, 1978; Endicott, Cohen, Nee et al., 1979) deals with the results of a study involving 175 newly admitted male and female inpatients with families who were randomly assigned to three groups: standard inpatient care followed by outpatient care (N=63); brief hospitalisation followed by day care and discharge to outpatients (N=61); and brief hospitalisation followed only by discharge to outpatients (N=51). The design of the study was such that any patient readmitted during the 2-year period after the index admission was again given the initially assigned treatment. Day patients were treated on the inpatient service. There was no separate day care programme or staff. The main difference between day patients and inpatients was that the former went home at night and during weekends. Over half the sample was aged under 35 years and came from social classes IV or V, and two-thirds had a diagnosis of schizophrenia. Measurements of the patients' psychopathology, social role functioning, the family 'burden', and the costs of treatment were made at entry, after 3 and 6 months, and at 6-monthly intervals up to 2 years after admission.

The average initial stay was 60 days for the standard group, and 11 days for both the brief groups. There was no statistically significant difference in readmission rates, but there was a significant difference among the groups in the average number of days of inpatient care received during the 2 years of the study: 115 days for the standard group, 47 days for the group which received day care, and 27 days for the brief group which was merely discharged to outpatients after admission. The day care group spent an average of 43 days in day care over the 2 years, but only about half those eligible made use of the facility.

The results showed that there were few differences among the treatment groups on any measures of psychiatric and social disorder, either the inpatients or their families. When differences did occur they tended to favour the brief groups. A crude analysis of the costs involved showed that brief hospitalisation followed by either day care or outpatient care was less expensive than standard hospitalisation, in respect of both hospital costs and costs to the patients' families.

Looking at the problem from another point of view, Linn, Caffey, Klett et al. (1979) investigated 162 male cases of schizophrenia receiving maintenance anti-psychotic drugs who were referred for day treatment at the time of discharge from ten Veterans' Administration hospitals. The patients were randomly assigned to day treatment plus drugs or outpatient drug management alone. In this study day care staff interviewed patients prior to randomisation in order to exclude patients who were thought to be inappropriate for referral to day care. Eighty-eight per cent of the day care subjects attended for a full day. Ten per cent attended less than 3 days a month. The most frequently prescribed treatments were social and recreational activities, group therapy, individual counselling, occupational therapy, and work counselling and training. Follow-up lasted 2 years, and six 6-monthly assessments were made of the patients' psychiatric symptoms, social functioning, attitudes, time spent out of hospital in the community, and the costs of care. A series of process variables about the day treatment centres were also recorded 6-monthly.

The results showed that all centres seemed to improve the patients' social functioning. Six of the centres were found to delay relapse significantly, to reduce symptoms, and to change some of the patients' attitudes. Centres with good results were characterised by the provision of more occupational therapy and a sustained non-threatening environment. Those with poor results were characterised by more psychologist and social work staffing hours, group psychotherapy, more family counselling, and a high patient turnover. The costs of treatment for the two treatment groups were not significantly different, though only patients' day and hospital costs were entered into the calculations. Overall, the centres with poor results were associated with significantly higher costs than centres with good results, a finding which was probably related to the excess of professional staff hours noted above.

(c) Individual goals and organisation of services

These findings lead directly on to two further considerations: the neglected and related issues of how to define individual patients' goals in day treatment, and of how to structure the professional organisation of day treatment to achieve many different objectives. There are, in fact, few reports of day treatment programmes which have linked a detailed assessment of each patient's physical, psychological, and social needs with particular therapeutic strategies. Falloon and Talbot (1982) describe such an exercise in which patients' goals were specified in terms of objectively defined behaviour to be achieved on or before a given time. Good outcome was associated with high levels of participation by patients in defining their own goals. In addition, goals concerned with social and vocational behaviour were achieved more frequently than those concerning symptoms and intrapersonal matters. A similar type of 'goal attainment scaling' was used in a comparative evaluation of 56 randomly selected patients who attended two day hospitals (Austin, Lieberman, King and DeRisi, 1976). One used a token economy system and behavioural and educational methods, concentrating on everyday coping and social skills, and occupational therapy. The other was more eclectic and made use of a therapeutic community approach involving community meetings, and group and individual psychotherapy. After intake, patients were followed up by interview at 3 and 6 months, and by telephone at 2 years. Although the results were not conclusive, the patients who attended the behavioural–educational programme attained more of their therapeutic aims.

This general theme, that certain professional and treatment practices may be of greater benefit than others in terms of staff–patient relationships and therapeutic outcome, was also raised by a study which investigated aspects of the organisation, management practices, and social interactions in four local authority day centres (Shepherd and Richardson, 1979). The centres were found to differ markedly. Nevertheless, a principal finding was that patient-oriented management attitudes were found to be correlated with a more personal approach to patients' problems and an emotionally warmer quality of personal interaction. However, high patient orientation, high rates of personal problem-solving and warm accepting staff–patient relationships are particularly desirable only if they can be shown to improve patients' functioning: and, as the authors point out, there is a need for more studies of the effects of variations in organisational and therapeutic methods on staff and patient behaviour.

(d) Conclusions

Satisfactory answers to the crucial questions about day treatment for patients with severe psychiatric disorder have not been forthcoming. There is now a need for clinicians and research workers to place more emphasis on the individual assessment and treatment of patients, and on the reliable and valid measurement of therapeutic outcome. Furthermore, the kind of detailed local inquiry that will be required to solve the current disorder is demonstrated by a survey of long-term users of community psychiatric services in Camberwell (Wing, 1982). This provided detailed information on the demographic, social and clinical characteristics of patients; the practices of day and residential units in relation to the social behaviour of attenders; the role of relatives; and the needs for, and the deployment of, services. Even so, as Wing (1982) emphasises, such exploratory studies cannot provide final answers. They may, however, suggest where changes in existing services should be made, and this in turn should lead to further evaluative studies in a cycle of planning and evaluation (Wing, 1972).

At this present state of knowledge it is concluded that day treatment lacks adequate evidence for its efficacy, and should be employed only under conditions that will permit rigorous experimental evaluation of its effectiveness in the management of specific disorders. It would seem likely that many specific patient needs for mental health management can be met most efficiently within an ambulatory care setting where the duration and intensity of intervention strategies is extended beyond that offered in the 50-minute outpatient consultation. Research is urgently required to determine the precise contingencies of methods that maximise the efficacy of day treatment.

11.5 COMMUNITY-BASED 24-HOUR CARE

The application of effective management of acute episodes of mental disorders usually involves the provision of (a) a calm, supportive interpersonal environment; (b) psychological treatment strategies for coping with distressing symptoms, and (c) the judicious application of specific pharmacological interventions. There is no evidence to suggest that this management is more effective when administered within the confines of a hospital ward than in other suitable locations in the community. On the contrary, in all controlled studies that have compared hospital care of acute episodes with community alternatives, the community location has proven of equal or greater effectiveness

225

(Mosher and Keith, 1980).

Dick (1982) provided an excellent summary of the concept of an acute 'bed' in psychiatry.

The function of the bed in psychiatry differs from the function of the bed in other branches of medicine. It is usually the place where the patient sleeps at night during a period of treatment or observation. It is not as important as the treatment place although it clearly has a role in assessment, observation, investigation, necessary separation and, at times, of acute illness, containment. However, the majority of psychiatrically troubled people are best sleeping in their own surroundings and family structure and not in exile.

It is sometimes argued that hospital-based observations of behaviour are an essential part of the assessment of a mental illness. While certain endocrine, neurological or other specialised medical assessments may require a controlled environment of the kind most readily found within a structured medical ward, Bennett (1982) raises the important issue that valid behavioural observation is best conducted in naturalistic settings, seldom found in psychiatric wards:

If we are interested in assessing the role behaviour of a patient, that behaviour can only be assessed by observing the person in a realistic situation; it may be a work situation, a family situation or a social situation. It is quite clear that observation in the ward of a traditional hospital is not satisfactory. Nor is it adequate to make an assessment using tests, questionnaires or structured interviews. Real life situations can be introduced into hospital though this is rarely done.

The question of providing cost-effective management of acute episodes of mental disorders seems not so much whether there are adequate alternatives to psychiatric hospital wards, but rather, are hospital wards the appropriate setting to manage acute mental illness in the first place? Arguments about staff convenience and containment of dangerous individuals are not medical considerations *per se* and should not be of primary concern. High levels of violence in psychiatric wards, where many disturbed, often defenceless individuals are threatened by violent patients, does little to suggest that mental hospitals provide an effective alternative to other community settings who attempt to deal with this problem. Mendel, Houle and Osman (1980) argue that herding disturbed, potentially violent individuals into a group-living setting is a foolhardy exercise likely to enhance the risk of violence rather than reduce it. However, it is notable that violent acts committed by patients in mental hospitals upon other patients (and often upon staff) are generally condoned by the staff, thereby setting a dangerous double-standard that effectively permits persons admitted to mental hospitals (whether mentally ill or not) to engage in violent acts outside the judicial guidelines set by the community for the remainder of its members. Such behaviour of persons labelled mentally disturbed extends beyond the confines of the hospital ward and contributes to the fears expressed by the community towards community-based management of mental disorders (Stein and Diamond, 1985). We would argue that first and foremost it is the business of the mental health providers to establish programmes that enable the most effective management of mental disorders, and that social and economic considerations are of concern only where they interfere with this process. It is hypothesised that the most effective management plan for a patient is also the most socially and economically viable plan from a long-term perspective.

Several model programmes have demonstrated the enhanced effectiveness of home-based management for acute episodes of mental illness. The best evaluation of such a method has been provided by Stein and Test (1980) in Madison, Wisconsin, and the replications by Fenton, Tessier, Struenig et al. (1982) and Hoult, Reynolds, Charbonneau-Powis et al. (1983). These studies provide an excellent model for the comprehensive evaluation of mental health services. Stein and Test (1980) established a programme called Training in Community Living, that aimed to manage patients in community settings who would otherwise have been admitted to a psychiatric ward. Their initial approach (since modified) was to remove patients from family living and treat them in boarding homes and independent apartment settings where they were encouraged to continue their daily activities with the assistance of mental health professionals, who provided 24-hour home-based care where necessary. Psychiatric and psychological assessment was made in the community setting and drug treatment provided by the mental health team. In addition to support to families and landladies, extensive liaison with police, social agencies, and even local businesses and shops was provided with immediate assistance being given to handle any problems that arose. Care was taken to encourage all persons in the community to treat mentally disordered persons in the same way as any other persons; in particular, to take a firm line on any anti-social behaviour. Management extended beyond dealing with the acute episode to comprehensive training of the patient in social, vocational and leisure activities and in the prevention of further episodes.

A controlled study of 130 cases randomly assigned to the community or hospital-based services examined the clinical, social and economic benefits of this approach. After 14 months of management the home-based programme showed a greatly reduced need for hospital care and reduced clinical and social morbidity (Stein and Test, 1980; Test and Stein, 1980).

The home-based programme proved more costly than the more traditional hospital-based programme, but the economic benefits to the patient and community far exceeded the additional costs (Weisbrod, Test and Stein, 1980). This finding points out a major problem in the establishment of effective alternatives to hospital care. They may prove more expensive in terms of direct costs to the health authorities, but they may reduce the costs to other public agencies such as social services, police and employment services. An economic analysis must include all sources of costs and benefits in this manner.

The two major limitations of these approaches are the relative lack of involvement of families and the long-term dependence on the mental health professionals. The behaviour therapy studies of family management and social skills training, discussed in the earlier section of this chapter that concerned outpatient services, suggest that a problem-oriented, self-help model may provide more effective long-term management. In contrast to the rapid deterioration noted when the TLC services were phased out (Stein and Test, 1980), the behavioural approaches appeared to continue to demonstrate effectiveness long after active training was completed (Falloon, 1985; Wallace and Liberman, 1985).

In summary, therefore, there is compelling evidence from well-controlled research evaluations to suggest that the intensive care facilities of the inpatient hospital service can be more efficiently provided in a home-based setting with benefits to patient, family and the community. Such an approach provides a framework for long-term rehabilitation that merges traditionally distinct inpatient, day-patient and outpatient services into a cohesive, continuous process that maximises support from community caregivers. In Britain these resources include the extensive primary care services and local authority social services.

In almost all these controlled evaluations of mental health treatment methods long-term outcome has been limited to no more than 2 years. This contrasts with the 5-year outcome standard employed in other medical fields. Clearly there is a need for longer studies of mental health care despite all the difficulties that such evaluation presents.

Cost-efficiency

In this era of diminishing financial resources there is an increasing demand to examine new services from an economic standpoint. The ideal new service will utilise the same, or less, resources to meet more of the community needs than the service it replaces. Two approaches to examining this issue are cost-benefit analysis and cost-effectiveness analysis. Both derive from the economic principles of alternative costs and diminishing returns.

In a cost-benefit analysis all costs and benefits are given monetary values. The results can then be expressed in terms of pounds spent per pound benefit. In the health field, however, the benefits that accrue cannot always be expressed in monetary terms. They often concern the quality of life of patients and their caregivers. In these instances a better approach is to compare costs with the effectiveness of the service to achieve clinical and social benefits that can be quantified numerically on standardised rating scales. In this way less tangible benefits, such as enhanced interpersonal functioning or reduced family stress, can be assessed in terms of the costs of interventions required to achieve such gains. This approach is termed a cost-effectiveness analysis. Of course, it may be argued that these benefits will eventually translate into monetary benefits when patients and their caregivers experience less disability and as a result obtain jobs more readily, or improve their jobs, at the same time reducing their need for intensive professional and community support. Such life changes are more likely to occur in the short term where effective treatment is provided at the earliest stage in the development of the disorder, prior to the social breakdown frequently associated with established major mental illness. With disorders of long duration rehabilitation may be a longer process, extending over several years. Thus an economic analysis should be tailored to the expected level of gains for the population that is being studied.

Economic studies of health care services are a relatively new field, and as yet there is no agreement on the procedures for conducting such evaluations (Goldberg and Jones, 1980). The direct costs of a mental health service are relatively easy to estimate if restricted to the time spent by professional staff in face-to-face contact with the index patient. However, such cost estimates are only applicable to the treatment of minor uncomplicated neurotic conditions (e.g. Ginsberg and Marks, 1977). The management of major mental illness necessitates care provided by a team of professionals, including general practitioners, social services and other community agencies such as the police. Institutional care provided for groups of patients, e.g. hospital wards, day hospitals, or hostels provides further complexity in the derivation of costs. This includes the problem of costing the under-utilisation of such resources. A hospital ward, fully staffed, will cost the same when completely filled with patients as when it is almost empty. Thus, the cost *per patient* will vary according to the level of utilisation. Costs based upon the assumption of constant full utilisation of such a resource will underestimate the true cost per patient.

Where patients are cared for at home, the direct costs of 24-hour professional care may be reduced. However, the costs may be considerable when family members are required to take leave from work or make other special provisions for home-based care. No provision has yet been made for the compensation of relatives for home-based programmes of acute care. It is crucial that all significant costs are estimated, not merely those accrued by the mental health service.

Several studies have compared the economics of community-based programmes. Murphy and Datel (1976) compared the costs of community care and hospital management of chronically mentally ill and mentally retarded patients. The cost of community care included housing and subsistence, while the benefits included the wages received from jobs and the savings from not having to maintain an institutional care facility. This study concluded that over a 10-year period the monetary benefits of community management would exceed the costs that were estimated for the same period.

Paul and Lentz (1977) used a cost-effectiveness analysis in their controlled comparison of three programmes of care for long-stay psychiatric patients. A behaviour therapy programme was more effective at achieving sustained community tenure than milieu therapy or the standard hospital programme. Furthermore, it was the least expensive. During more than 4 years that the project was operating 90 per cent of the patients were successfully rehoused in the community at one-third of the cost of both the standard hospital programme and the milieu programme. Reductions in the need for professional staff and medication accounted for the major savings. This analysis did not examine the indirect costs, benefits or savings associated with community-based management. It appeared likely that these costs would increase the advantages associated with the sophisticated rehabilitative methods employed in this study.

Fenton et al. (1982) compared the costs of home-based and hospital-based management of acute mental illness during the first year of treatment in a controlled trial. The home treatment proved more cost-efficient. The cost to the families from time lost from work and out-of-pocket expenses was small, although the emotional stress was high in both conditions. The main costs involved professional time in outpatient and inpatient services. The cost of managing schizophrenia was greater than for other disorders. Once again, no attempt was made to estimate the benefits that may have accrued from effective home-based care.

Cardin, McGill and Falloon (1985) found that a programme of family management was more than twice as cost-efficient as more traditional patient-based community management of schizophrenia. In the first year of the programme direct and indirect costs were 19 per cent less with family management. The savings that accrued would have enabled 22 per cent more patients to be managed for the same cost as the traditional methods, with additional resources becoming available in subsequent years.

The most sophisticated economic analysis of a community mental health service to date was conducted by Weisbrod et al. (1980). They employed a cost-benefit analysis in their controlled study of home-based management of mental illness.

Monetary values were applied to all direct and indirect services, as well as to societal costs, such as law enforcement for patients' misdemeanours or loss of family income. The monetary benefits that accrued from competitive and sheltered employment and the reductions in clinical, social and family morbidity were assessed. The community-based approach produced greater monetary benefits, but at a slightly greater cost than the hospital-based approach. The added monetary benefits were three times greater than the additional costs. In addition, as discussed earlier, the non-monetary benefits of reduced clinical, social and family morbidity favoured the community approach.

11.6 CONCLUSIONS

It is evident that the technology of economic evaluation of mental health services is in a relatively early stage of development. However, several excellent studies have been conducted. These studies tend to support the conclusion that community-based programmes tend to make more efficient use of resources, thereby having the potential to meet more of the needs of the community. Studies of this nature require careful planning and implementation to ensure that all the costs and benefits to the community are comprehensively assessed. To date the methods refined by Weisbrod (1981) represent the current state of the art, but there is considerable room for improvements, especially in the difficult area of quantifying improvements in the quality of life in economic terms. Until this can be done the focus of these studies will remain on reducing the utilisation of the most expensive resources, such as hospital and outpatient services.

11.7 THE BUCKINGHAM PROJECT: A HOME-BASED MENTAL HEALTH SERVICE

A model mental health service for a rapidly growing rural community of between 30,000 and 40,000 has been developed in the North Aylesbury Vale. This service has been based on the principle that the comprehensive mental health needs of a community can be most efficiently met by providing assertive professional support to the existing generalist services provided by families, primary health care teams and social agencies. This contrasts with the traditional hospital-based specialist services where extensive resources are provided only for the most severely disturbed patients, who are usually removed from the care of their community resources.

Three teams of four or five nurses are trained to work as specialists within the three primary care teams in the area. They are deployed on a 24-hour basis with each team to conduct assessments and provide specialist management at the request of general practitioners, community nurses, social services and police. Assessment and treatment is usually provided at the patient's home, although there is a small foster-home scheme and admission to the GP-managed community hospital is occasionally sought.

The mental health teams are led by a senior nurse therapist with training in behaviour therapy methods for managing psychiatric and neurotic disorders. A 2-year training programme is conducted for all nurses entering the service. The mental health teams are supported by a full-time panel of consultants, including a consultant psychiatrist, a senior registrar, a psychologist, an occupational therapist and a social worker, as well as two administrative secretaries. This consultant panel meets weekly at each health centre, and is readily available to provide additional support to the mental health nurses. At all times the general practitioner remains the primary manager of the case and mental health records are integrated with the patient's general medical records. Patients are assessed at their convenience, and initial consultation is provided on the day of referral, although in some non-urgent cases this may be brief.

Cost-effective management approaches are employed throughout. These include: cognitive/behavioural treatment of anxiety and depressive disorders (with antidepressant drugs in cases with 'endogenous' features); family stress management combined with pharmacotherapy for schizophrenia and bipolar disorders; and behavioural stress management approaches for adjustment disorders, including the stress of chronic physical illness. The emphasis is on early detection of major mental illness and immediate intensive treatment.

Patients who do not respond to early intervention, or who remain undetected until their conditions are severe, are managed by extensive care at home. The nursing and consultant staff are employed to provide a level of care similar to that provided in an excellent inpatient setting.

Patients with major handicaps and their caregivers are provided with individualised psychosocial rehabilitation programmes on a long-term basis. This may include extensive assistance from the occupational therapist and psychologist, as well as continual reassessment of medication needs.

These methods are being evaluated in terms of their effectiveness in reducing clinical, social and family morbidity in a defined community (i.e. all patients registered with the 15 GPs in the area). It is hypothesised that a reduced prevalence of chronic mental disorders and associated social handicaps will be observed once the service has been fully deployed, and that this model will prove a highly cost-efficient way to meet the mental health needs of a community. The early signs appear extremely promising, although definitive conclusions will have to await long-term evaluation.

REFERENCES

Ambelas, A. (1986) 'Life Events and Mania — A Special Relationship?', *British Journal of Psychiatry*, *15*, pp. 235-40

Austin, N.K., Liberman, R.P., King, L.W. and DeRisi, W.J. (1976) 'A Comparative Evaluation of Two Day Hospitals. Goal Attainment Scaling of Behaviour Therapy vs Milieu Therapy', *Journal of Nervous and Mental Disease*, *163*, pp. 253-62

Beck, A.T. (1986) 'The current status of cognitive therapy'. Lecture to British Association of Behavioural Psychotherapy, Central Branch, Oxford

Bellack, A.S., Herson, M. and Himmelhoch, J.M. (1983) 'A Comparison of Social-skills Training, Pharmacotherapy and Psychotherapy for Depression', *Behaviour Research and Therapy*, *21*, pp. 101-7

Bennett, D. (1982) 'What Direction for Psychiatric Day Centres?', in *MIND Yearbook 1981/82*, National Association for Mental Health, London

Brown, G.W. and Harris, T. (1978) *Social Origins of Depression: A Study of Psychiatric Disorder in Women*, Tavistock, London

Burgess, J. (1983/84) (personal communication) 'A survey of admissions to hospital from the North Aylesbury Vale'

Cardin, V.A., McGill, C.W. and Falloon, I.R.H. (1985) 'An Economic Analysis: Costs, Benefits and Effectiveness', in I.R.H. Falloon (ed.), *Family Management of Schizophrenia*, Johns Hopkins University Press, Baltimore, Md.

Carpenter, W.T., Stephens, J.H. and Rey, A.C. (1982) 'Early Intervention vs Continuous Pharmacotherapy of Schizophrenia', *Psychopharmacology Bulletin*, *18*, pp. 21-3

Corney, R.H. (1984) 'The Effectiveness of Attached Social Workers in the Management of Depressed Female Patients in General Practice', *Psychological Medicine*, Monograph supplement 6

Davis, J.M., Schaffer, C.B., Killian, G.A., Kinard, C. and Chan, C. (1980) 'Important Issues in the Drug Treatment of Schizophrenia', *Schizophrenia Bulletin*, 6, pp. 70-87

Dick, D. (1982) 'Alternatives for the care of the mentally ill in Surrey', keynote address to Surrey Area Health Authority Seminar, Brighton

Dilling, H. and Weyrerer, S. (1984) 'Prevalence of Mental Disorders in the Small Town Rural Region of Traunstein (Upper Bavaria)', *Acta Psychiatrica Scandinavica*, 69, pp. 60-79

Endicott, J., Herz, M.I. and Gibbon, M. (1978) 'Brief versus Standard Hospitalisation: the Differential Costs', *American Journal of Psychiatry*, 135, pp. 707-12

Endicott, J., Cohen, J., Nee, J., Fleiss, J.L. and Herz, M.I. (1979) 'Brief versus Standard Hospitalisation: For Whom?', *Archives of General Psychiatry*, 36, pp. 706-12

Falloon, I.R.H. (1985) *Family Management of Schizophrenia: A Study of the Clinical, Social, Family and Economic Benefits*, Johns Hopkins University Press, Baltimore, Md.

Falloon, I.R.H. and Liberman, R.P. (1983) 'Interactions between Drug and Psychosocial Therapy in Schizophrenia', *Schizophrenia Bulletin*, 9, pp. 543-54

Falloon, I.R.H. and Talbot, R.E. (1982) 'Achieving the Goals of Day Treatment', *Journal of Nervous and Mental Disease*, 170, pp. 279-85

Falloon, I.R.H., Hole, V., Pembleton, T. and Norris, L. (In press) 'Behavioural Family Interventions in the Management of Manic-depressive Disorders', in J.F. Clarkin, G. Haas and I.D. Glick (eds), *Family Intervention in Affective Illness*, Guilford Press, New York

Fenton, F.R., Tessier, L., Struenig, E.L., Smith, F.A. and Benoit, C. (1982) *Home and Hospital Psychiatric Treatment*, Croom Helm, London

Follette, W.C. and Jacobson, N.S. (1987) 'Behavioral Marital Therapy in the Treatment of Depressive Disorders', in I.R.H. Falloon, (ed.), *Handbook of Behavioral Family Therapy*, Guilford Press, New York

Gibbons, J.L., Jennings, C. and Wing, J.K. (eds) (1981) *Psychiatric Care in 8 Register Areas: Statistics from Eight Psychiatric Case Registers in Great Britain, 1976-1981*, University of Southampton, Southampton

Ginsberg, G and Marks, I. (1977) 'Costs and Benefits of Behavioural Psychotherapy: a Pilot Study of Neurotics Treated by Nurse Therapists', *Psychological Medicine*, 7, 685-700

Goldberg, D. and Huxley, P. (1980) *Mental Illness in the Community: The Pathway to Psychiatric Care*, Tavistock, London and New York

Goldberg, D. and Jones, D. (1980) 'The Costs and Benefits of Psychiatric Care', in L.N. Robins, P.J. Clayton and J.K. Wing (eds). *The Social Consequences of Psychiatric Illness*, Brunner/Mazel, New York

Goldstein, M.J., Rodnick, E.H., Evans, J.R., May, P.R. and Steinberg, M. (1978) 'Drug and Family Therapy in the Aftercare Treatment of Acute Schizophrenia', *Archives of General Psychiatry*, *35*, 1169-77

Hafner, R.J. and Marks, I.M. (1976) 'Exposure in vivo of Agoraphobics: Contributions of Diazepam, Group Exposure and Anxiety Evocation', *Psychological Medicine*, *6*, pp. 71-88

Herz, M.I., Endicott, J. and Spitzer, R.L. (1975) 'Brief Hospitalisation of Patients with Families; Initial Results', *American Journal of Psychiatry*, *132*, pp. 413-18

Herz, M.I., Endicott, J. and Spitzer, R.L. (1976) 'Brief versus Standard Hospitalisation: the Families', *American Journal of Psychiatry*, *133*, pp. 795-801

Herz, M.I., Endicott, J. and Spitzer, R.L. (1977) 'Brief Hospitalisation: a Two-year Follow-up', *American Journal of Psychiatry*, *134*, pp. 502-7

Herz, M.I., Endicott, J. and Gibbon, M. (1979) 'Brief Hospitalisation: Two-year Follow-up', *Archives of General Psychiatry*, *36*, pp. 701-5

Hogarty, G.E. (1984) 'Aftercare Treatment of Schizophrenia', in *Schizophrenia*, Update Publications, London

Hoult, J., Reynolds, I., Charbonneau-Powis, M., Weeks, P. and Briggs, J. (1983) 'Psychiatric Hospital versus Community Treatment: the Results of a Randomised Trial', *Australian and New Zealand Journal of Psychiatry*, *17*, pp. 160-7

Johnstone, E.C., Owens, D.G.C., Gold, A., Crow, T.J. and MacMillan, J.F. (1984) 'Schizophrenic Patients Discharged from Hospital — a Follow-up Study', *British Journal of Psychiatry*, *145*, pp. 586-90

Kane, J. (1983) 'Low Dose Medication Strategies in the Maintenance Treatment of Schizophrenia', *Schizophrenia Bulletin*, *9*, 29-33

Leff, J., Kuipers, L., Berkowitz, R., Eberlein-Vries, R. and Sturgeon, D. (1982) 'A Controlled Trial of Social Intervention in the Families of Schizophrenic Patients', *British Journal of Psychiatry*, *141*, pp. 121-34

Linn, M.W., Caffey, E.M., Klett, J., Hogarty, G.E. and Lamb, H.R. (1979) 'Day Treatment and Psychotropic Drugs in the Aftercare of Schizophrenic Patients: A Veterans Administrative Cooperative Study', *Archives of General Psychiatry*, *36*, pp. 1055-66

Marks, I.M. (1981) *Cure and Care of Neuroses*, Wiley, New York

Marks, I.M. (1985) 'Controlled Trial of Psychiatric Nurse Therapists in Primary Care', *British Medical Journal*, *290*, pp. 1181-4

Mendel, W., Houle, J. and Osman, S. (1980) 'Mainstreaming: An Approach to the Treatment of Chronically and Severely Mentally Ill Patients in the Community', *Hillside Journal of Clinical Psychiatry*, *2*, pp. 95-128

Miklowitz, D.J., Goldstein, M.J., Nuechterlein, K.H., Snyder, K.S. and Doane, J.A. (In press), 'The family and the course of recent onset mania'

Milne, D.L. (1986) *Training Behaviour Therapists: Methods, Evaluation and Implementation with Parents, Nurses and Teachers*, Croom Helm, London/Brookline Books, Cambridge, Mass.

Mosher, L.R. and Keith, S.J. (1980) 'Psychosocial Treatment: Individual, Group, Family and Community Support Approaches', *Schizophrenia Bulletin*, 6, pp. 10-41

Murphy, J.G. and Datel, W.E. (1976) 'A Cost-benefit Analysis of Community versus Institutional Living', *Hospital and Community Psychiatry*, 27, pp. 165-70

Parkes, C. (1978) 'On the Use of Psychiatric Resources for Indirect Service', *Bulletin, Royal College of Psychiatrists*, pp. 29-33

Paul, G.L. and Lentz, R.J. (1977) *Psychosocial Treatment of the Chronic Mental Patient*, Harvard University Press, Cambridge, Mass.

Paykel, E.S., Mangen, S.P., Griffith, J.H. and Burns, T.P. (1982) 'Community Psychiatric Nursing for Neurotic Patients: A Controlled Trial, *British Journal of Psychiatry*, 140, pp. 573-81

Prien, R.F. (1984) 'Long-term Maintenance Pharmacotherapy in Recurrent and Chronic Affective Disorders', in M. Mirabi (ed.), *The Chronically Mentally Ill: Research and Services*, Spectrum, New York

Raeburn, J.M. and Seymour, F.W. (1977) 'Planning and Evaluating Community Health and Related Projects: A Systems Approach', *New Zealand Medical Journal*, 86, pp. 188-90

Regier, D.A., Burke, J.D., Manderscheid, R.W. and Burns, B.J. (1985) 'The Chronically Mentally Ill in Primary Care' *Psychological Medicine*, 15, 265-73

Regier, D.A., Myers, J.K., Kramer, M., Robins, L.N., Blazer, D.G., Hough, R.L. Eaton, W.W. and Locke, B.Z. (1984) 'The NIMH Epidemiological Catchment Area Program: Historical Context, Major Objectives and Study Population Characteristics', *Archives of General Psychiatry*, 41, 934-41

Reibel, S. and Herz, M.I. (1976) 'Limitations of Brief Hospital Treatment', *American Journal of Psychiatry*, 133, 518-21

Schooler, N.R. and Keith, S.J. (1983) 'Treatment Strategies in Schizophrenia', Research Proposal, National Institute of Mental Health, Rockville, Md.

Shepherd, G. and Richardson, A. (1979) 'Organisation and Interaction in Psychiatric Day Centres', *Psychological Medicine*, 9, 573-9

Shepherd, M., Cooper, B., Brown, A.C. and Kalton, G. (1966) *Psychiatric Illness in General Practice*, Oxford University Press, Oxford and New York

Shepherd, M., Wilkinson, G. and Williams, P. (1986) *Mental Illness in Primary Care Settings*, Tavistock Publications, London and New York

Sloane, R.B., Staples, F.R., Cristol, A.H., Yorkston, N.J. and Whipple, K. (1975) *Psychotherapy versus Behavior Therapy*, Harvard University Press, New York

Stein, L.I. and Diamond, R.J. (1985) 'The Chronic Mentally Ill and the Criminal Justice System: When to Call the Police', *Hospital and Community Psychiatry*, 36, 271-4

Stein, L.I. and Test, M.A. (1980) 'An alternative to Mental Hospital Treatment: I. Conceptual Model, Treatment Program and Clinical

Evaluation', *Archives of General Psychiatry*, *37*, 392-9

Strathdee, G. and Williams, P. (1984) 'A Survey of Psychiatrists in Primary Care: the Silent Growth of a New Service', *Journal of the Royal College of General Practitioners*, *34*, 615-18

Test, M.A. and Stein, L.I. (1980) 'Alternative to Mental Hospital Treatment: III. Social Cost', *Archives of General Psychiatry*, *37*, 409-12

Tyrer, P. (1984) 'Psychiatric Clinics in General Practice: An Extension of Community Care', *British Journal of Psychiatry*, *145*, 9-14

Tyrer, P., Seivewright, N. and Wollerton, S. (1984) 'General Practice Psychiatric Clinics: Impact on Psychiatric Services', *British Journal of Psychiatry*, *145*, 15-19

Vaughn, C.E. and Leff, J.P. (1976) 'The Influence of Family and Social Factors on the Course of Psychiatric Illness: A Comparison of Schizophrenic and Depressed Neurotic Patients', *British Journal of Psychiatry*, *129*, 125-37

Wallace, C.J. and Liberman, R.P. (1985) 'Social Skills Training for Patients with Schizophrenia: A Controlled Clinical Trial', *Psychiatry Research*, *15*, 239-47

Weisbrod, B.A. (1981) 'Benefit Cost Analysis of a Controlled Experiment: Treating the Mentally Ill', *Journal of Human Resources*, *16*, 523-48

Weisbrod, B.A., Test, M.A. and Stein, L.I. (1980) 'An Alternative to Mental Hospital Treatment: II. Economic Benefit, Cost Analysis', *Archives of General Psychiatry*, *37*, 400-5

Weissman, M.M. Prusoff, B.A., Dimascio, A., Neu, C., Goklaney, M. and Klerman, G.L. (1979) 'The Efficacy of Drugs and Psychotherapy in the Treatment of Acute Depression', *American Journal of Psychiatry*, *136*, 555-8

Wilkinson, G. (1984) 'Day Care for Patients with Psychiatric Disorders', *British Medical Journal*, *288*, 1710-12

Wilkinson, G. (1985) *Mental Health Practices in Primary Care Settings*, Tavistock, London and New York

Wilkinson, G. and Freeman, H. (1986) *The Provision of Mental Health Services in Britain: The Way Ahead*, Gaskell, London.

Wing, J.K. (1968) 'Social Treatments of Mental Illness', in M. Shepherd and D.L. Davies (eds), *Studies of Psychiatry*, Oxford University Press, London

Wing, J.K. (1972) 'Principles of Evaluation', in J.K. Wing and A.M. Hailey (eds), *Evaluating a Community Psychiatric Service: the Camberwell Register*, Oxford University Press, London

Wing, J.K. (ed.) (1982) 'Long-term Community Care: Experience in a London Borough', *Psychological Medicine*, *12* (Monograph supplement 2)

World Health Organization (In preparation), 'Cross-cultural differences in the 5-year course and outcome of patients with an initial diagnosis of schizophrenia

Zitrin, C.M., Klein, D.F., Woerner, M.G. and Ross, D.C. (1983) 'Treatment of Phobias. I: Comparison of imipramine hydrochloride and placebo', *Archives of General Psychiatry*, *40*, 125-38

12

Evaluation in Social Work

Eileen Gambrill

EDITOR'S INTRODUCTION

Our final chapter takes the social work perspective on mental health service evaluation. Dr Gambrill's approach is to review the broad range of methods that have been adopted to date, including single-case studies, experimental and quasi-experimental research designs, and programme evaluations. Examples are provided for each of these methods and they are illustrated with data from the social work literature.

Eileen Gambrill also discusses the need for evaluation and some of the prevailing beliefs about the whole process, including the view that evaluation trivialises client concerns and that it interferes with the therapeutic relationship. In short, she suggests that the term evaluation is emotionally loaded, with a history of confrontations between academic and practitioner, not to mention between social workers of differing therapeutic orientation. However, she concludes with some constructive suggestions for minimising confrontation and facilitating participation in evaluation. They include clarifying beliefs, supporting and shaping existing skills, and providing research tools.

Social workers provide a substantial portion of the personal social services both in Britain and the United States. In the United States for example, the bulk of community mental health services are offered by social workers. Evaluation within social work encompasses a broad array of activities including programme evaluation, single-case studies, and experimental and quasi-experimental projects designed to explore the effectiveness of certain kinds of intervention programmes. Some writers in the field of evaluation also include other endeavours under the rubric of evaluation, such as needs assessment (e.g. Rossi and Freeman, 1985). Examples of evaluation in social work are described in this chapter to provide readers with illustrations of the potential for evaluation in social work settings. The role of evaluation in social work is first discussed below. Examples of evaluation research are then presented, and guidelines for encouraging evaluation efforts discussed.

12.1 THE ROLE OF EVALUATION IN SOCIAL WORK

Lack of attention to accountability by social workers has been a major concern in the social work literature (e.g. Briar, 1974). The need for, and optimal qualities of, evaluation have long been a topic of concern within social work (Reid and Smith, 1981). Positions in this debate range from one viewing social work as an art and evaluation in any rigorous fashion as therefore unsuitable, to one viewing social work as an applied endeavour the effectiveness of which can be improved by clear identification of outcomes and careful evaluation of progress. The latter position views evaluation as both an ethical and practical matter; ethical in offering consumers a choice of intervention methods that have been found to be effective in relation to given outcomes as well as feedback concerning degree of progress (or its lack) and practical in terms of gaining ongoing information concerning the effects of intervention allowing timely alteration of intervention plans and continued motivation of clients.

Studies of the effectiveness of social work include areas of delinquency prevention, child guidance cases, marital counselling, acting-out behaviour of young boys, multi-problem families, protective services to the aged, and families on welfare (Fischer, 1976; Reid and Hanrahan, 1982). Some studies suggest that the effects of social work are not necessarily positive; that deterioration may occur. For example, a study of protective services to elderly people found that clients receiving social work services had higher death rates than did clients not receiving such services (Blenkner, Bloom and Nielsen, 1971). Discussions of evaluation in the social work literature often have a confrontational tone in which researchers and academics are pitted against practitioners. This stance has been unfortunate; it has helped to scare off practitioners who otherwise might have been encouraged to evaluate their practice more carefully. The increased interest in single-case designs and increased sensitivity on the part of researchers to concerns and realities of day-to-day practice have helped to break down this polarised view. Most social workers would agree that evaluation is important. An interest in evaluation on the part of practitioners has been encouraged by requirements of funding agencies and increase in peer review. Thus, most social workers do care about evaluation. Reasons include a concern about clients in terms of offering helpful service; an interest in acquiring and maintaining access to funds; avoidance of malpractice suits; and showing up well on peer reviews. The National Association of Social Workers Code of Ethics (1980) calls on social workers to evaluate their practice as do many social work tests (e.g. Gambrill, 1983; Fischer, 1978; Reid, 1978; Pinkston, Levitt, Green *et al.*, 1982). Peer review requires evaluation of service. It is not that social workers disagree that evaluation is important. *How* and *what* to evaluate are the issues. For example, 95 per cent of a group of British social workers (*N*=25) said that they evaluated their work with clients. However, many could not identify clear progress indicators. What may be wanting in methods used include the following:

(1) use of subjective measures (e.g. self-report) alone– uncomplemented by objective measures (e.g. observation in real-life settings);
(2) vague rather than clear measures;
(3) pre–post rather than continuous tracking of progress;
(4) social worker's opinions concerning progress rather than, or not complemented by, feedback from clients and significant others;
(5) use of only process (what was done) or outcome (what happened) measures rather than both.

Both self-report and objective measures of progress should be gathered in view of the fact that neither kind of measure may offer accurate data (Wolf, 1978) and because discrepancies between subjective and objective data can offer helpful clinical information. For example, such differences may reveal that objective measures selected are not of relevance to clients. Timing of evaluation is also important. Pre–post measures do not provide the day-to-day feedback offered by on-going monitoring of degree of progress. How long should positive effects last? Answers to this question will be influenced by one's theory concerning behaviour. Ideally, follow-up of client's progress would be a routine part of an agency's practice. For an example of a self-report instrument used to gather follow-up data, see Beck and Jones, 1980 (see also Mutschler, 1979).

(a) Beliefs about evaluation

Some social workers believe that evaluation trivialises human concerns; that it can only be done in a mechanical way that either demeans people and/or focuses on relatively trivial changes; changes unrelated to richly textured presenting problems. Some believe that it interferes with clients' rights to privacy. Other social workers believe that evaluation is boring; that it will simply make their work more onerous for negligible gains. Many correctly believe that there's no such thing as an objective measure, but incorrectly equate this belief with the false belief that all measures yield equally accurate information about progress (see Figure 12.1).

Figure 12.1: Beliefs about evaluation

1. Trivialises client concerns
2. Is boring
3. All measures distort the real world equally
4. Interferes with offering service to clients (takes too much time; is too intrusive)
5. Interferes with the therapeutic relationship
6. Is only feasible when using behavioural methods
7. Arbitrary time periods must be used

Profoundly different views about *what* and *how* to evaluate practice coupled with the purpose of evaluation (to answer questions such as: was my work effective?) make this subject a touchy one. Some writers in the general area of evaluation stress this point. Patton (1981), for example, who is one of the most prolific writers about evaluation, may start a workshop by asking participants to free-associate about what the term evaluation means; what fears, preconceptions, expectations, and beliefs are associated with evaluation. 'When you hear the word evaluation, what comes to mind? (p. 97). Another method he uses is placing a number of objects, such as paper bags and cups, in a pile on a table and asking each person to select an object and use that item to make a statement about evaluation. One person wrote:

> This empty grocery bag is symbolic of my feelings about evaluation. When I think about our programme being evaluated I want to find someplace to hide and I can put this empty bag over my head so that nobody can see me and I can't see anything else, and it gives me at least the feeling that I'm able to hide. [She puts the bag over her head.] (p. 98).

This illustrates how the word evaluation is loaded with emotional reactions. Not only may progress achieved be reviewed, the explanations for such progress may also be examined and found wanting. Emotional reactions, lack of familiarity with relevant empirical studies, and a failure to examine critically the premises as well as the form of arguments used to explain or justify actions taken, all conspire to maintain faulty beliefs about evaluation.

(b) Options for evaluation

Options for evaluation depend in part on resources available. Most social workers (if not all) have the potential option of learning how to carry out single-case designs as a part of their routine practice, using the information provided to make informed clinical decisions. Use of single-case studies is limited by the degree of interest in and familiarity with such methods, and by availability of required skills such as identification of specific relevant objectives and selection of valid, feasible, progress indicators. Inability of an agency to provide immediate service to all clients, natural breaks occasioned by illness and vacations, and inability to intervene in all areas at once in complicated cases, provide opportunities to conduct single-case designs that offer more rigour compared to AB designs which include a baseline phase followed by an intervention phase (Gambrill and Barth, 1980).

12.2 SINGLE-CASE DESIGNS

Recent years have seen an increase among social workers in use of single-case designs (Bloom and Fisher, 1982; Jayaratne and Levy, 1979). These designs offer information related to the following clinical questions: (1) Is intervention working? (2) Is one intervention better than another? (3) Is it more effective to combine two or more procedures? (4) What level of intervention is best? and (5) Was intervention responsible for change? (Hayes, 1981). The potential utility of single-case studies in social work settings is considered quite problematic by some (Thomas, 1978) and more promising by others (Gambrill and Barth, 1980). There is no doubt that use of such designs requires certain key skills such as identification of specific relevant objectives and clear, sensitive, feasible progress indicators, and there is also no doubt that social workers typically do not acquire such skills in the course of their formal education or agency-based training.

It is not true that use of a single-case design requires a baseline phase; degree of progress can be tracked even if intervention is initiated without such a phase. What is required is clear description of outcomes desired, and multiple measurement points within each phase. It is true that different questions can be answered depending on whether baseline data are available. A view of the research enterprise as a continuum ranging from designs that are exploratory in nature and offer tentative data concerning the effects of a procedure to designs that permit inferences about the causal effects of interventions permits an optimistic view of the utility of a range of single-case designs (Gambrill and Bath, 1980). The collection of information within designs that do not permit causal inference does not necessarily interfere with practice, and in many if not most cases it can facilitate practice in terms of allowing timely alteration of plans and maintenance of client motivation. Restricting activities to single-case study designs that are rigorous overlooks important contributions to the development of knowledge that social workers can make within less rigorous designs.

The AB design (baseline followed by intervention) provides a weak basis for believing that a given intervention was responsible for observed changes. However, replication across clients or occasions decreases vulnerability to some types of confounding effects. For example, successful repetition of an AB design using the same intervention across different clients with similar problems (such as parent training with abusive parents) can provide information on the generality of findings. Although such replications do not resolve questions about the role of specific components of intervention, these questions can be explored later in a context in which research issues are given priority.

Information concerning goals achieved by all social workers in an agency can be reviewed by administrators to determine the effectiveness of service with given kinds of problems/client mixes. Review of outcomes achieved by individual practitioners can be used to offer feedback (e.g. Bolin and Kivens, 1974). Examples of the use of single-case designs in community settings are given in the next section.

(a) Examples of single-case designs

Evaluation is a routine part of the family approach to the care of the elderly described by Pinkston and Linsk (1984). Family members as well as clients are involved in recording information that allows on-going evaluation of progress as illustrated in the example below.

Mrs Banks, a 67-year-old divorcee, was hospitalised because of 'paranoid behaviours' which took place in the home of her daughter. These included accusations, swearing, shouting, refusal to take medication, and reported hallucinations. She was said to be illiterate and had a diagnosis of 'stable dementia' and memory problems. Mrs Banks had a son, a daughter, and a grand-daughter. Assessment indicated that social deprivation, not the initial referral problems of bizarre behaviours, was the most serious problem. Mrs Banks said that she would like to go out to a club or organisation once a week, go to the store two or three times a week, and go for daily walks. An increase in community contacts was the long-range intervention goal for Mrs Banks.

It was agreed that Mrs Banks be located in her own apartment. Family contracts were drawn up identifying tasks related to agreed-on goals. These also provided feedback to family members for task completion. A family behaviour record was used by family members to record frequency of

245

appropriate talking, swearing, and talking to herself. The family also recorded frequency of contacts with visitors, and visits outside of the home. By the end of the third week all tasks were completed and an apartment was rented. Talking to herself decreased to almost zero and appropriate conversation increased moderately. After the move Mrs Banks kept track of visitors and phone calls. Both visitors per week and telephone calls increased (see Figure 12.2). Visits with her daughter increased to two or three a week, visits with her son occurred weekly, and talks with her grand-daughter and daughter took place daily. This pattern of family contact was maintained for 3 years and Mrs Banks continued to live in her own apartment.

Monitoring of progress served an important function in this case, as in the other examples presented below. 'Without such monitoring, Mrs Banks' level of reinforcement and activity might have become so low that new behaviour problems could have emerged in an effort to attract some social attention' (Pinkston and Linsk, 1984, p. 64).

Single-case designs were used to evaluate the effectiveness of a systematic decision-making procedure in working with biological parents and their children who were in foster care (see description of the Alameda Project in a later section). An example of data collected in relation to one multi-problem family is described below (Stein, Gambrill and Wiltse, 1978).

Steven W., 9½ years, was declared a dependent of the court, and criminal charges were filed against his father for abuse. Mrs W. was not involved in the incident. No court action was taken in regard to the other four children at home. Both parents said that they wished to have their son returned to their home and Steven said he would like to return home. A problem profile was completed, and the worker and clients agreed to begin working on three problems. Reducing the father's drinking was seen as the most important issue by both parents. According to Mrs W., when Mr W. drank in the evenings he retreated from the problems created by the children, which increased Mrs W.'s responsibilities and frustration. She stated that she had no free time to herself, and resented the restrictions on her and the overall responsibility for running the house. Both drinking and frustration in

Figure 12.2: Mrs Banks's weekly frequency of visitors and telephone calls

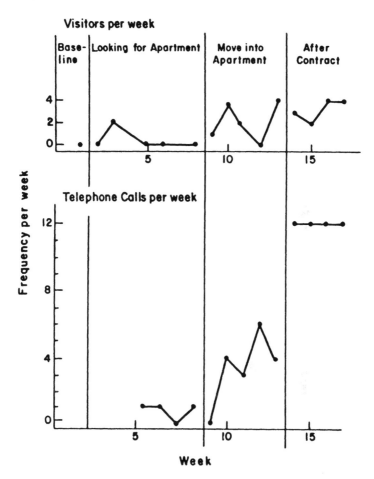

Source: Pinkston and Linsk, 1984, p. 63.

relation to the children's lack of chore completion were considered to be related to the abuse, and assessment focused on these areas.

The worker suggested that a contract be formed with the objective of restoring Steven to his parents' home contingent on reducing the father's drinking and increasing the mother's free time and the children's completion of chores. Since Mr W. did not show any effects of drinking until after three drinks, it was decided that he could have two drinks per day. Regular visits with Steven were planned. Intervention plans were designed to decrease alcohol use and to increase chore completion and free time for Mrs W. (see Stein *et al.*, 1978; Stein and Gambrill, 1983, for more detailed descriptions).

Sixty days from the time of contract signing, Mr W.'s drinking was reduced from a baseline of $6^{1}/_{2}$ drinks per day to $3^{1}/_{2}$ drinks per day. He was earning his agreed-on 1 hour of free time and engaging in nightly discussions with Mrs W. about his work. Mrs W.'s free time increased beyond the objective of 2 hours per week to 4 hours. The parents had negotiated the latter increase on their own, and both were satisfied with this arrangement (see Figures 12.3 and 12.4). Visits with Steven had occurred according to schedule, and no problems were observed by the worker or reported by the parents. The parents were inconsistent in maintaining records of chore behaviour of their children. Information they did collect showed that at the beginning of the programme the children were earning an average of four points per day, and that this had increased by approximately two points per child per day.

Ninety days from contract signing, Mr W.'s drinking decreased to zero drinks per day, and Mrs W.'s free time had increased to 8 hours per week. As agreed, Mr W. assumed child-care responsibilities during these additional hours. The parents reported that the children's compliance with household responsibilities increased; however, they did not maintain records in this area.

Steven returned to his parents' home as specified in the contract. For the first 2 months following restoration the worker maintained bi-weekly in-person contact and alternate-week telephone contact with the family. No problems were observed, nor were any reported by the parents. The worker remained with this case for 90 additional days of follow-up. Steven was still reported to fight on occasion with his siblings, but not to an extent that was considered to be a problem. The court dependency was dismissed.

Both individual and group data are used to evaluate the effectiveness of a parent training programme designed by Dangel and Polster (1984). Objectives are taught in short units and mastery criteria are identified for each unit. Criteria are

Figure 12.3: Average number of alcoholic drinks consumed per day by Mr W.

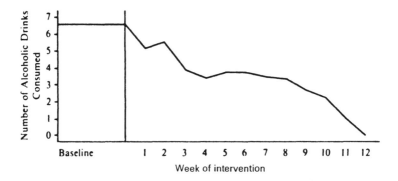

Figure 12.4: Hours of free time per week for Mrs W.

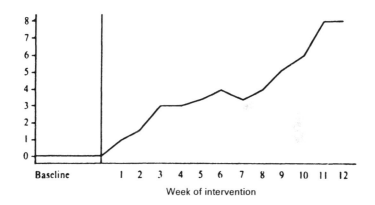

Source: Stein *et al.*, 1978, p. 237, copyright © 1978 Praeger Publishers.

cumulative across lessons. Parents receive immediate quantitative feedback following each training session in relation to the number of times they use each skill, as well as qualitative feedback in the form of comments describing their skills. The programme is self-paced so that parents can progress at their own speed. Parents complete 'checkouts' after each lesson and parenting behaviour is also observed at home. This offers the parent an opportunity to demonstrate mastery of skills in real-

249

life settings. Activities observed vary, and have included getting ready for bed, cleaning the bathroom, and watching television. The parent receives immediate feedback using a specially designed checkout sheet for each skill, such as praise and attention. The total number of behaviours observed during the observation period is compared with the criteria number. Immediate feedback is given after each observation period. 'For example, one statement is made about passing the lesson, two statements about use of skills for the current lesson, two about the use of skills from the previous lesson, one about the importance of practise, and zero to two suggestions for improvement' (p. 178).

Over 2,000 families have participated in this parent training programme since 1978. A variety of evaluation methods have been used to review results including checklists, scales, inventories, role plays, in-home observation, and parent self-report. Checkouts (described above) provide multiple opportunities to evaluate the results of specific phases throughout the programme. Observation of video-tapes of parent–child interaction is also used to evaluate effectiveness. Data are collected on eleven categories of parent behaviour and eight categories of child behaviour. Parent behaviours include praise, suggestive praise, rewards and privileges, removing rewards and privileges, directions, repeated directions, time out, attention, spanking, physical abuse, and parent–child interaction. Child behaviours include appropriate behaviour, misbehaviour, compliance, fighting, back-talking, household chores, temper tantrums, and whining. Four evaluation studies of this programme involving 62 families showed that positive consequences increased by 153 per cent, attention to inappropriate behaviour decreased by 44 per cent and interaction increased by 42 per cent. Inappropriate behaviour decreased for 86 per cent of the children; the mean percentage decrease was 44 per cent. Parent satisfaction with the programme was high. All parents, poor, wealthy, minority, non-minority, single-parent, and two-parent demonstrated mastery of the skills. Parents reported that they found the programme helpful and enjoyed it.

This programme, like the others described in this section, illustrates the clinical utility of single-case designs in which data are collected concerning progress or its lack on an on-going basis. The requirements of this design mesh closely with requirements of planned intervention based on observation of results achieved. The programmes described illustrate the attention to baseline levels in the design of intervention plans, as well as how data collected on individual clients can be cumulated to gain an overview of the usefulness of a programme with many clients. There is thus a close relationship between evaluation at the case level and evaluation at the agency or administrative level.

(b) Exploring within-session changes

Often, effects are expected within a session. Changes can be measured before and after the session as well as at points in between. Data collected provide useful information as to whether an intervention is successful in the office setting. Thyer and Curtis (1983) report the use of in-session evaluation with a 26-year-old housewife who had a severe fear of frogs which interfered considerably in her life. A behavioural approach test was used to assess her initial repertoire as well as to monitor progress. Heartbeat and subjective anxiety was determined within each treatment session for different approach behaviours. The client's reactions during the first and sixth sessions are shown in Figures 12.5 and 12.6. Degree of approach behaviour in real-life settings based on observation and/or self-report can be used to supplement in-session data.

12.3 EVALUATION IN GROUP SETTINGS

Social workers have been in the forefront of evaluating the effectiveness of interventions offered in groups. Examples of populations and areas addressed include battering men (Edleson et al., 1985), pregnant teenagers (Blythe, Gilchrist and Schinke, 1981), elderly clients (Toseland, Sherman and Bliven, 1981), smoking (Schinke, Gilchrist and Snow, 1985), and depression (Berlin, 1985).

Both self-report and observation measures were used to evaluate the effectiveness of a communication skills workshop for couples (Rose, 1977). Three couples met in a group for six sessions. Evaluation measures were gathered a week before training as well as 1 week and 6 weeks following training. Self-

Figure 12.5: First treatment session pre–post behavioural approach tests

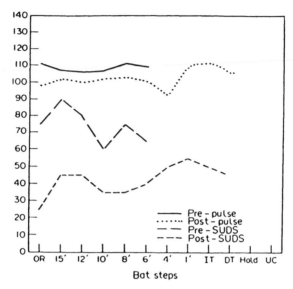

Source: Thyer and Curtis, 1983, p. 313.

Figure 12.6: Sixth treatment session pre–post behavioural approach tests

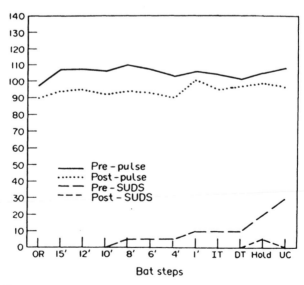

Source: Thyer and Curtis, 1983, p. 314.

report measures were used to assess communication effectiveness and marital satisfaction, and interaction in two conflict situations was observed. Gains were found on all measures, and clients reported that the programme was useful. A number of evaluation studies conducted by social workers emphasise prevention. The effectiveness of group training in decision-making and interpersonal skills to prevent unwanted adolescent pregnancy was explored by Blythe and her colleagues (Blythe et al., 1981). Nineteen high school students were randomly assigned to treatment and control groups. Students in the intervention group met with a male/female team of graduate social work students for 14 semi-weekly 1-hour sessions. Intervention included didactic presentation, discussion, role-playing, modelling, coaching, feedback, and social reinforcement. Subjects were encouraged to use the information provided to plan and review the consequences of actions. A quiz was given to the students at the beginning of each session to evaluate retention of material. Teenagers receiving group training answered more questions and scored significantly better on tasks essential to effective decision-making in social relationships; they identified more potential obstacles and were better able to describe problems from different perspectives. Participants in the group intervention made more eye contact, refused more unreasonable demands and made more requests for behaviour changes in others' behaviour as determined from a review of video-tapes of role-playing in stressful interpersonal situations. Their perception of the usefulness of the project was very positive. Follow-up data collected 3 and 6 months after the last session showed that teenagers who had received training had greater commitment to postponing pregnancy, used birth control more often, and had greater reliance on more effective birth control methods compared to control group members.

Berlin (1985) explored the effectiveness of relapse prevention procedures in maintaining low levels of self-criticism among a clinical sample of self-critical women. Women were selected from a pool who applied to a community mental health centre for help with self-criticism or related problems such as low self-esteem or depression. Self-criticism themes concerned deficient performance, achievement, and work effort; personal attributes, such as physical appearance; and perceived deficiencies in comparison to others or feeling devalued by others. Most women (64 per cent) linked their self-criticism to underlying perfectionist standards. A pre-test–post-test comparison group design was used, in which subjects were randomly assigned to one of two conditions: standard cognitive-behavioural intervention and relapse prevention intervention. Each group was further divided into two small groups of five or six members each. Co-leader teams were assigned to one standard and one relapse prevention group in order to distribute leaders across different groups. Women in both groups participated in eight group treatment sessions and four individual assessment sessions: pre-test, post-test, and 2- and 6-month follow-up.

The standard intervention was designed to reduce negative self-attribution by altering unrealistic expectations, increasing competence, and replacing negative evaluations with more helpful self-statements. There was no systematic attempt to avert relapse. Subjects in the relapse-prevention group also received instruction on maintaining gains. This consisted of identifying high-risk situations, developing and rehearsing coping strategies, and clarifying reluctance to cope actively with given problem situations.

Measures used included a situational coping test, a perfectionism scale, and self-report measures of depression and self-esteem. The Situational Coping Test (SCT) consisted of 12 tape-recorded descriptions of high-risk situations to which women described their imagined responses (see Berlin, 1985, for a detailed description of how these situations were selected). An example of an item is: 'Imagine that you've had a really hard week. You haven't finished very many of the projects you wanted to be done with by now, the house is a mess, and you're feeling generally run-down and tired. What are you thinking to yourself in response to this situation?' Subjects also rated the relevance of each item to their own lives. Responses to vignettes were scored according to frequency of self-critical responses, frequency of positive coping responses, response latency, and overall outcome favourability. Coping responses were identified as discrete thoughts expressing or implying efforts or plans to change situations or alter stressful reactions. Self-monitoring was used to determine daily frequency of self-criticism during the first and last treatment weeks and in the week preceding each follow-up interview. Women were given a small booklet of forms to record criticisms. Hourly periods were described across the top of each, and reasons for self-criticism were listed along the side from top to bottom. During every hour in a 12-hour period, women reviewed the previous hour and recorded any self-criticism in the cell corresponding to the appropriate hour and reason.

Relapse was defined as deterioration of improvement from post-test to the 2-month or 6-month follow-up. Women in both conditions showed improvements in their responses to the SCT and maintained these improvements 6 months following the end of treatment. Women in the relapse condition did not show superior maintenance effects except for greater decreases in self-criticism from the pre-test to the 6-month follow-up. Frequencies of self-criticisms decreased and frequencies of positive coping increased in both conditions from pre- to post-test and were maintained through the follow-up period. The relapse prevention condition had greater pre- to post-test decreases in self-criticism and greater decreases from pre-test to the final follow-up. Women in both conditions reported fewer self-criticisms and maintained these reductions through the follow-up period. Depression scores decreased in both conditions. In summary, women in both conditions showed decreases in self-criticism and related problems at post-test and tended to maintain improvements. Failure to find between-group differences may have been due to a number of factors, including the brevity of the intervention period or use of different group leaders.

These findings offer additional support for the value of cognitive–behavioural strategies in decreasing depression. There were no controls for non-specific effects (e.g. being in a group, attention, encouragement) since the design compared two intervention procedures. A design involving two intervention procedures may be more feasible in some settings compared to a design including an attention-placebo group or a waiting-list group.

(a) Exploring changes within group sessions

Changes in behaviour during group sessions can also be evaluated. For example, Figure 12.7 shows changes in member-to-member and leader-to-member interactions over sessions (Rose, 1977, p. 49).

Figure 12.7: Direction of interaction

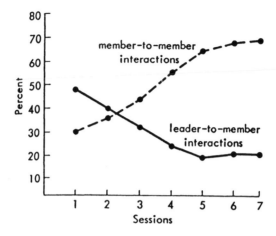

Source: Rose, 1977, p. 49.

12.4 FIELD EXPERIMENTS

This option requires more resources and greater up-front planning compared to the use of single-case designs. The aim of field experiments is to explore the effectiveness of one or more intervention methods in relation to a desired outcome. Initial phases require establishing a constructive working relationship with agency staff. The more closely staff are involved in these early phases, and the more helpful they anticipate the outcomes will be, the smoother early as well as later phases will be.

There are a number of conditions under which field experiments may be desirable to agencies. One is when the objectives of an agency change. For example, one precursor to the Alameda Project (described below) was the dwindling supply of adoptable infants to a large adoption agency and the subsequent need to deal with older children coming into foster care. This change increased interest on the part of a private agency (the Children's Home Society) in funding the Alameda Project which was conducted in co-ordination with a large public agency. This project illustrates combining resources of a public and private agency towards an aim of mutual interest.

(a) The Alameda Project

The goals of the Alameda Project were to develop and test methods to: (a) increase parental participation in making decisions for the future living arrangements of their children; and (b) compare the effects of services offered within a social–behavioural framework with regular agency practice (see Stein *et al.*, 1978, for further details). The project was conducted over a period of 2 years with a 1 year follow-up to evaluate the stability of placements made. Criteria for selection of cases were: (a) the child was under 16 years of age; (b) the child was in a foster home; (c) the child had at least one parent living in the county; and (d) a decision for the child's future living arrangements had not yet been made. The initial caseload was volunteered by workers participating in the project; new cases were randomly assigned. A total of 428 children were included in the experimental ($N=227$) and control units ($N=201$). Problems associated with child maltreatment included depression, alcohol and drug abuse, poor parenting skills, lack of material resources, marital conflict, and problems with relatives. Project workers were trained in behavioural methods including assessment, intervention, and contracting.

By the end of the project a permanent plan had been accomplished or was in progress for 79 per cent of the children served by experimental unit staff compared to 40 per cent of those served by control workers. Differences between groups were significant ($p<0.001$) for each type of plan. A greater percentage of children in the experimental units as compared with the control units was returned or were to be returned to their biological parents, were adopted or in the adoptive process, were assigned a legal guardian or were waiting for court dates for consideration of such assignment. A smaller percentage of children in the experimental units was headed for long-term foster care.

Length of time in care predicted outcome for experimental unit children: 60 per cent of those in care for less than 1 year were returned to their own homes. Restoration decreased as length of time in care increased. Whether biological parents signed written case plans was predictive of ongoing parental involvement. Of the families who signed agreements, 70 per cent worked to their chosen goal of reunification; of families who did not sign agreements, only 16 per cent had their children returned to their care. Achievement of the goals of a signed working agreement was predictable 57 per cent of the time. Follow-up took place 1 year after the project ended. Disruption of placement occurred for only one child in the experimental and one child in the control unit, both of whom had been returned to their biological parents during the project.

This project demonstrated that experimental services were more effective than regular agency practice in achieving permanent placements for children in foster care. Single-case designs were used to track progress on an on-going basis in individual cases (see prior section on single-case designs for an example).

Social work offers many possibilities for field experiments. Limitations imposed by money or agency decisions may require compromises in the rigour of evaluation procedures used resulting in quasi-experimental designs (Cook and Campbell, 1979).

12.5 GOAL-ATTAINMENT SCALING

Goal-attainment scaling, which was originally developed for use in community mental health programmes, offers another way to assess progress (Kiresuk and Sherman, 1968). This procedure involves identifying a series of objectives in terms of desirability. The first step is identification of major areas in which change is desired. A second step involves selection of a variable in each area that will serve as a measure of success. For example, interest in work could be assessed in terms of specific client statements in relation to work. A third step requires the identification of a series of outcome levels in each area based on the variables selected in the second step. The expected level of outcome is the one considered most likely, and outcomes that represent more and less than expected are included above and below the expected outcome. Progress can be assessed in terms of outcomes attained, arriving at a goal-attainment change score (Kiresuk and Garwick, 1975; p. 394). Baseline levels can be indicated on the scale by placing an asterisk in the cell corresponding to this value.

12.6 NEEDS ASSESSMENT

Another kind of evaluation research that social workers can carry out with limited resources is that of needs assessments. A needs assessment can provide answers to questions such as: what needs do people have for specific kinds of services? How well do current services meet specific needs? What barriers exist to use of services and how can these be removed? Need may be assessed in a variety of ways including 'felt need' (people are asked whether they need a service) and 'expressed need' (use of a service). Each has advantages and disadvantages in terms of offering valid information (Bradshaw, 1972; Ross and Freeman, 1985).

12.7 PROGRAMME EVALUATION

A major theme of this chapter is that options for evaluation within social work exist both at the individual case and agency level, and that data collected at the case level can be of value at the agency-wide level in assessing effect achieved. Evaluations differ considerably in their rigour; in the kinds of answers provided about effectiveness and the role of particular intervention procedures in relation to outcomes achieved. The kind of evaluation possible will depend in part on the resources available both in terms of money and of skills. Programme evaluation often does not involve experimental manipulation of an independent variable. Hypotheses may not be explicitly stated, and if they are they usually derive more from the goals of the programme rather than from a theory (Tripodi, Fellin and Meyer, 1969). Random distribution of clients to different intervention conditions is often not possible, and agency objectives are often vague, making it difficult to identify agreed-on and relevant progress indicators.

There is a rich literature in the area of programme evaluation — some of which is very sensitive to important considerations such as ensuring that agency staff are involved in the process of evaluation and that evaluation be user-focused; that is, designed to be of value to staff (Patton, 1978). If it is not, staff may interpose an endless series of obstacles to evaluation efforts. Even if such an effect can be circumvented, staff may not make use of results if they are not involved in the evaluation process. All too often these sound guidelines are not followed; that is, evaluation is designed by people external to an agency with little or no input by agency staff, with the all-too-frequent outcome that data discovered are not used. In such cases the question should be raised, 'Who benefits?' Certainly not the recipients of service.

12.8 ENCOURAGING SOCIAL WORKERS TO EVALUATE THEIR PRACTICE

It's really not a great mystery why social workers don't evaluate their practice more rigorously; why, for example, they often use fuzzy, subjective indicators of progress. Required conceptual frameworks, knowledge, and skills as well as cues and incentives to maintain careful evaluation of practice are typically absent. The greater the fear about evaluation (what will be expected; what will be revealed) and the less the familiarity with related empirical literature, the easier it will be for social workers to accept uncritically false statements about evaluation.

The number of social workers who use progress indicators that are more, rather than less, accurate can be increased by paying as much attention to diffusing new evaluation methods as to developing them. Material that describes helpful strategies for encouraging people to explore new methods can be drawn on towards this end. There are four important sources of literature that can be used to advantage. These concern (1) diffusion of innovations; (2) evaluation; (3) relationships between behaviour and environmental factors; and (4) requisites for effective training programmes. Steps that can be taken to encourage evaluation efforts are described below.

Coax out beliefs about evaluation. People are not likely to change their behaviour in ways that conflict with important beliefs. An exploration of the meanings associated with evaluation will yield clues about why evaluation is such a touchy topic. Beliefs that interfere with evaluation should be addressed, and beliefs that encourage related efforts encouraged. Information about what social workers believe will be helpful in selecting methods for encouraging them to take a look at other frameworks. Attention to beliefs highlights the importance of a broad view of the usefulness of evaluation; this broad view includes helping social workers to: (1) clarify their beliefs about evaluation; (2) identify and review their ideologies; (3) clarify and review practice goals; and (4) discover different ways to track progress.

Enhance clear thinking skills. Knowledge about judgemental strategies will help social workers to use strategies that result in accurate accounts. Sources such as *Straight and Crooked Thinking: 39 Dishonest Tricks of Debate* (Thouless, 1974) can be used to familiarise social workers with sources of errors and remedies for these (see also Nisbett and Ross, 1980). Knowledge about the effects of a particular setting, such as case conferences on the accuracy of judgement, will be helpful (see, for example, Meehl, 1973).

Consider user goals. Some writers in the field of evaluation have been so struck with the lack of attention to what individual practitioners hope to get out of evaluating their work that they highlight this by using titles such as *User-Focused Evaluation* (Patton, 1978); making the point that evaluation should serve the goals of practitioners.

Support available competencies. Trainers often find out what social workers can't do; that is, conduct a mini-needs assessment or deficiency analysis unaccompanied by an assets analysis (finding out what they *can* do in relation to evaluation). A deficiency description is not likely to encourage risk-taking or to lower fears, nor does it offer opportunities to support skills that already exist. One innovative method Patton (1981) uses to reveal to participants that they already know a great deal about evaluation is to ask them to sabotage an evaluation plan that is presented. This exercise reveals a surprising variety of helpful skills that practitioners already have, and offers opportunities to support these assets.

Identify intermediate steps. Initial repertoires may be far removed from what is desired both in terms of motivational characteristics as well as accompanying skills. Planned behaviour change usually requires progressing through a series of intermediate steps tailored to initial individual competencies. Important steps such as clarifying ideologies and beliefs, as well as available skill levels and interests, are often ignored in efforts to encourage evaluation. Evaluation of practice is integrally related to assessment and intervention. How are goals selected? What will be considered signs of progress? A broad view of the usefulness of evaluation as separate from the accuracy of findings is critical to appreciating the value of intermediate steps.

Provide required knowledge and skills. It is unfair to expect social workers to evaluate their practice when they don't have the knowledge and skills to do so. Identifying clear objectives is an important related skill. Selection of objectives often requires high-quality assessment skills to select objectives that are not only specific, but that are also achievable and relevant to client concerns. Most social workers do not know how to set specific objectives. For example, 95 per cent of a sample of British social workers ($N=25$) said that they did set specific objectives, yet only 5 per cent could actually do so. This reveals yet another hurdle; many social workers think they do set clear objectives when in fact they do not. The belief that you are already doing something is a significant obstacle to improving skills in an area.

Setting clear objectives requires a number of assessment skills such as selecting wisely from among different sources of assessment information and decreasing or avoiding conditions that may reduce the accuracy of data collected. Social workers who do not have needed skills often reject careful evaluation because they say it only works with 'trivial' objectives; the objectives they may select may indeed be 'trivial' because of a lack of assessment skills.

Provision of knowledge and skills will require well-designed training programmes which consider initial repertoires and individual learning styles, and which take advantage of what is known about the requisities of effective training programmes (Argyris, 1982; Gagne, 1977). Ideally, the effects of training programmes should be evaluated in terms of competencies acquired and client outcomes attained by staff.

Provide required tools. Keeping up with available information about how to offer effective services is a problem for professionals. Making sure social workers have access to helpful assessment tools for self-monitoring and observation by trained personnel will encourage evaluation of practice (see for example Hudson, 1982 and Bellack and Hersen, 1987).

Arrange supportive cues and incentives. Follow-up studies of students trained in use of single-case studies show that such skills do not necessarily continue to be used on-the-job (e.g. Richey, Blythe and Berlin, in press). Attention should be devoted to arranging cues and incentives that will support behaviours related to evaluation. This will involve 'up-front' planning including involvement of agency personnel who have an interest in evaluation, description of cues and incentives currently provided in an agency in relation to evaluation efforts, and description of likely consequences of any changes (Mager and Pipe, 1970; Gambrill and Stein, 1983). What specific evaluation behaviours are or could be supported? What kinds of behaviours are or will be punished? What helpful cues can be provided?

Make written material more enticing. Material related to evaluation is often written in a dry, jargony manner that turns readers off. Use of a clear engaging writing style, together with use of case examples related to practice, will encourage practitioners to read helpful material.

Make careful evaluation easier. Evaluation can be made easier in a variety of ways, some of which have already been mentioned, such as having helpful tools available. If practitioners read more about evaluation they will be in a more informed position to select progress indicators that are relevant and sensitive to change. Computer processing of information will increase ease of evaluation both on the individual practitioner level as well as the agency level. For example, computer programs are available for scoring some inventories. Computerised information management systems will increase ready accessibility of agency-wide data concerning effects achieved. Evaluation options related to different kinds of desired outcomes can be stored on discs and viewed as needed. Interactive video-tape programs can be used to develop new social skills and to review progress along the way. Many of these suggestions will make evaluation fun, as well as helpful in offering valuable feedback.

Provide on-going consultation. On-going consultation is important in helping social workers to overcome obstacles and to provide support. Conditions required for maintenance of positive outcomes should be arranged based on empirical information about maintenance rather than assuming a 'train and hope' approach (Stokes and Baer, 1977).

12.9 INSURING THE FIDELITY OF ASSESSMENT AND INTERVENTION PROCEDURES

Ideally, evaluation should include clear descriptions of both process and outcome; that is, procedures used as well as outcomes achieved should be clearly described. All too often, studies do one or the other but not both. Lack of clear description of process is an unfortunate characteristic of a great deal of outcome research in social work. Studies that demonstrate that practitioners may not vary their behaviour as a function of methods used (Wodarski, Feldman and Pedi, 1974) highlight the importance of a description of what is done. Clear description of procedures used is important even when a supposedly agreed-upon method such as systematic desensitisation is used. Unless we are given a detailed description we really cannot judge the fidelity with which a procedure was offered, nor the match between the presenting problems and the wisdom of selecting a particular intervention method. More attention has recently been devoted to this problem (e.g. Derer, 1985; Nelson, 1985). Assessing the quality with which a procedure is offered is also of concern in evaluating diffusion efforts.

12.10 DEVELOPMENTAL RESEARCH AND DIFFUSION EFFORTS

Encouraging wider use of effective intervention methods is just as important as generating initial data concerning effectiveness. Diffusion of helpful methods has been relatively neglected in the field of interpersonal helping. That thoughtless diffusion efforts can have quite disastrous results has been illustrated (Rogers, 1983). Procedures found to be effective in successful demonstration projects are often not continued in the very counties in which they were evaluated, as was the case with the Alameda Project. Recently, additional attention has been devoted to a discussion of procedures that would encourage the use of, and generation of, practice-related research in an incremental fashion (e.g. Thomas, 1984: Rothman, 1980). The intent is to encourage immediate use of research concerning effectiveness as well as continued development of information in relation to given kinds of procedures and desired outcomes.

12.11 SUMMARY

Evaluation in social work encompasses a wide variety of activities including single-case designs, experimental and quasi-experimental studies, and programme evaluation which may make use of different kinds of research designs. Approaches to evaluation include acceptance of subjective self-reports of change which many would consider to be weak indicators, to the use of single-case designs involving tracking of specific progress indicators on an on-going basis as a routine part of practice. Personal, educational, and organisational factors influence the nature of evaluation efforts. Personal factors such as beliefs about social work practice (e.g. is it an art or a science?) and feelings of being threatened by finding out what is happening, pose obstacles to careful evaluation of progress. Organisations differ in the extent to which they provide tools, cues, and incentives that support evaluation. Social work education programmes typically do not prepare students to evaluate their practice.

A number of trends that influence social work, such as requirements by funding agencies to present data concerning effectiveness of services, as well as peer review, should encourage more careful evaluation efforts. Acceptance on the part of those who would like to encourage careful evaluation efforts of a broad perspective in relation to evaluation in terms of the many changes that may be required, will be helpful in encouraging social workers to take advantage of the feedback careful evaluation can provide.

REFERENCES

Argyris, C. (1982) *Reasoning, Learning and Action,* Jossey-Bass, San Francisco, Calif.

Beck, D.F. and Jones, M.A. (1980) *How to Conduct a Client Follow-up Study,* Family Service Association of America, New York

Bellack, A.S. and Hersen, M. (eds) (1987) *Behavioral Assessment: A Practical Handbook* (3rd edn), Pergamon, New York

Berlin, S. (1985), 'Maintaining Reduced Levels of Self-criticism through Relapse Prevention Treatment', *Social Work Research and Abstracts, 21,* pp. 21-33

Blenkner, M., Bloom, M. and Nielsen, M. (1971) 'A Research and Demonstration Project of Protective Services', *Social Casework, 52,* pp. 489-506

Bloom, M. and Fisher, J. (1982) *Evaluating Practice: Guidelines for the Accountable Professional,* Prentice-Hall, Englewood Cliffs, NJ

Blythe, B., Gilchrist, L.D. and Schinke, S.P. (1981) 'Pregnancy Prevention Groups for Adolescents', *Social Work, 26,* pp. 503-4

Bolin, D.C. and Kivens, L. (1974) 'Evaluation in a Community Mental Health Center, Huntsville, Alabama', *Evaluation, 2,* pp. 26-35

Bradshaw, J. (1972) 'The Concept of Social Need', *New Society, 30*, pp. 640-3

Briar, S. (1974) 'The Future of Social Work: An introduction', *Social Work, 19*, pp. 514-18

Cook, T.D. and Campbell, D.T. (1979) *Quasi-Experimentation: Design and Analysis For Field Settings*, Rand McNally, Chicago, Ill.

Dangel, R.F. and Polster, R.A. (1984) 'Winning! A Systematic Empirical Approach to Parent Training', in: R.F. Dangel and R.A. Polster (eds), *Parent Training: Foundations of Research and Practice*, Guilford Press, New York, pp. 162-201

Derer, K.R. (1985) 'Operational Specificity: Implications for Field-based Replications', *Journal of Behavior Therapy and Experimental Psychiatry, 16*, pp. 9-14

Edleson, J.L., Miller, D., Stone, G.W. and Chapman, D.G. (1985) 'Group Treatment for Men who Batter: A Multiple-baseline Evaluation', *Social Work Research and Abstracts, 21*, pp. 18-21

Fischer, J. (ed.) (1976) *The Effectiveness of Social Casework*, Charles C. Thomas, Springfield, Ill.

Fischer, J. (1978) *Effective Casework Practice: An Eclectic Approach*, McGraw-Hill, New York

Gagne, R.M. (1977) *The Conditions of Learning*, 3rd edn, Holt, Rinehart & Winston, New York

Gambrill, E.D. (1983) *Casework: A Competency Based Approach*, Prentice-Hall, Englewood Cliffs, NJ

Gambrill, E.D. and Barth, R.P. (1980) 'Single-case Study Designs Revisited', *Social Work Research and Abstracts, 16*, pp. 15-20

Gambrill, E. and Stein, T.J. (1983) *Supervision: A Decision-Making Approach*, Sage, Beverly Hills, Calif.

Hayes, S.C. (1981) 'Time Series Methodology and Empirical, Clinical Practice', *Journal of Consulting and Clinical Psychology, 49*, pp. 193-211

Hudson, W.W. (1982) *The Clinical Measurement Package: A Field Manual*, Dorsey Press, Homewood, Ill.

Jayaratne, S. and Levy, R.L. (1979) *Empirical Clinical Practice*, Columbia University Press, New York

Kiresuk, T.J. and Garwick, G. (1975) 'Basic Goal Attainment Scaling Procedures', in: B.R. Compton and B. Galaway (eds), *Social Work Processes*, Dorsey Press, Homewood, Ill.

Kiresuk, T.J. and Sherman, R.E. (1968) 'Goal Attainment Scaling: A General Method for Evaluating Comprehensive Community Mental Health Programs', *Community Mental Health Journal, 4*, pp. 447-53

Mager, R.F. and Pipe, P. (1970) *Analyzing Performance Problems*, Fearon Press, Belmont, Calif.

Meehl, P.L. (1973) 'Why I Do Not Attend Case Conferences', *Psychodiagnostic Papers*, University of Minnesota Press, Minneapolis, Minn.

Mutschler, E. (1979) 'Using Single-case Evaluation Procedures in a Family and Children's Service Agency: Integration of Practice and Research', *Journal of Social Service Research, 3*, pp. 115-34

Nelson, J.C. (1985) 'Verifying the Independent Variable in Single-subject Research', *Social Work Research and Abstracts, 21,* 3-8

Nisbett, R. and Ross, L. (1980) *Human Inference: Strategies and Shortcomings of Social Judgment,* Prentice-Hall, Englewood Cliffs, NJ

Patton, M.Q. (1978) *Utilization-focused Evaluation.* Sage, Beverly Hills, Calif.

Patton, M.Q. (1981) *Creative Evaluation,* Sage, Beverly Hills, Calif.

Patton, M.Q. (1982) *Practical Evaluation,* Sage, Beverly Hills, Calif.

Pinkston, E.M., Levitt, J.L., Green, G.R., Linsk, N.L. and Rzepnicki, T.L. (1983) *Effective Social Work Practice: Advanced Techniques For Behavioural Intervention With Individuals, Families, and Institutional Staff,* Jossey-Bass, San Francisco, Calif.

Pinkston, E.M. and Linsk, N.L. (1984) *Care of the Elderly: A Family Approach,* Pergamon, New York

Reid, W.J. (1978) *The Task-Centred System,* Columbia University Press, New York

Reid, W. and Hanrahan, P. (1982) 'Recent Evaluations of Social Work: Grounds for Optimism', *Social Work, 27,* 328-40

Reid, W.J. and Smith, A.D. (1981) *Research In Social Work,* Columbia University Press, New York

Richey, C.A., Blythe, B.J. and Berlin, S.B. (In press) 'Practitioner, Client and Agency Factors Associated with Maintenance of Single-case Evaluation', *Social Work Research and Abstracts*

Rogers, E.M. (1983) *Diffusion of Innovations,* 3rd edn, Free Press, New York

Rose, S.B. (1977). *Group Therapy: A Behavioral Approach,* Prentice-Hall, Englewood Cliffs, NJ

Rossi, P.H. and Freeman, H.E. (1985) *Evaluation: a systematic approach,* 3rd edn, Sage, Beverly Hills. Calif.

Rothman, J. (1980) *Using Research in Organizations: A Guide to Successful Application.* Sage, Beverly Hills, Ca.

Schinke, S.P., Gilchrist, L.D. and Snow, W.H. (1985)'Skills Intervention to Prevent Cigarette Smoking among Adolescents', *American Journal of Public Health, 75,* 665-7

Stokes, T.F. and Baer, D.M. (1977) 'An Implicit Technology of Generalisation', *Journal of Applied Behavior Analysis, 10,* 349-67

Thomas, E.J. (1978) 'Research and Service in Single-case Experimentation: Conflicts and Choice', *Social Work Research and Abstracts, 14,* 20-31

Thomas, E.J. (1984) *Designing Interventions for the Helping Professions,* Sage, Beverly Hills, Calif.

Thouless, R.H. (1974) *Straight and Crooked Thinking,* Pan Books, London

Toseland, R., Sherman, E. and Bliven, S. (1981) 'The Comparative Effectiveness of Two Group Work Approaches to the Development of Mutual Support Groups among the Elderly', *Social Work With Groups, 4,* 137-53

Thyer, B.A. and Curtis, G.C. (1983) 'The Repeated Pre-test, Post-test, Single-subject Experiment: A New Design for Empirical Clinical

Practice', *Journal of Behavior Therapy and Experimental Psychology*, *14*, 311-15

Tripodi, T., Fellin, P. and Meyer, H.J. (1969) *The Assessment of Social Research: Guidelines for the Use of Research in Social Work and Social Science*, Peacock, Itasca, Ill.

Wodarkski, J.S., Feldman, R.A. and Pedi, S.J. (1974) 'Objective Measurement of the Independent Variable: A Neglected Methodological Aspect in Community-based Behavioral Research', *Journal of Abnormal Child Psychology*, *2*, 239-44

Wolf, M.M. (1978) 'Social Validity: the Case for Subjective Measurement or How Applied Behavior analysis is Finding its Heart', *Journal of Applied Behavior Analysis*, *11*, 203-14

Part Three: Conclusion

13

Discussion and Conclusions

Derek Milne

We began this book by stating that its main aim was to help practitioners to conduct more and better research. This was then pursued by presenting a number of ideas and methods for evaluating our work, although additionally some so-called 'non-specific effect' may have been achieved through the enthusiasm of the contributors. We placed an emphasis upon the interests and procedures perceived as relevant by members of those working in the different mental health disciplines, so as to reduce the gap between where our professional training tends to leave off and our evaluation efforts begin.

It is clear from the contents of this book that mental health practitioners can address a diverse range of relevant questions and utilise a large number of different research methods in their search for answers to pressing service issues. If nothing else, this shows that it is possible to bridge the traditional scientist–practitioner gulf.

It is not, however, the intention here to review this research spectrum, but rather to pick out some of the salient points that have emerged in several chapters. Of particular interest are the ways in which practitioners actually engineer an evaluation study and the consequences they experience for this activity. Emerging from this is the issue of the structure of our mental health service and what model of service would be necessary if we are to increase the likelihood that more and better evaluation will take place in future.

13.1 ANTECEDENTS TO RESEARCH ACTIVITY

There are a number of general pressures on the practitioner to engage in research. They include a shift in public attitudes towards greater accountability on the part of the health services, more concern for patients' rights, a considerable restriction on financial resources, a growing demand for more efficient services and a trend toward community care. Although it should not be viewed as a panacea, systematic evaluation may offer practitioners a way of dealing with these pressures so as to preserve (or even develop) their services (Barlow, Hayes and Nelson, 1984).

In addition, individual practitioners may have their own reasons for undertaking research, ranging from a search for personal kudos to the pursuit of deeply held ethical beliefs about the best way to improve the quality of our care. Local characteristics such as a research tradition or simple opportunism may also contribute.

However, only a minority of practitioners actually engage in research, indicating that these pressures on their own are not the whole story. One factor which may go some of the way to explaining this state of affairs in terms of antecedent events is the nature of our training. There is now much greater scope for providing clinicians with relevant, relatively straightforward means of evaluating their work, as exemplified by developments in the single-subject case study (Hersen and Barlow, 1976). These methods can be addressed in training, so as to minimise the step between 'laboratory' and 'field', as advocated by Kazdin, Kratochwill and Vandenbos (1986). More fundamentally, training might change its emphasis towards what the late Don Bannister referred to as the 'invention' of professions. This entails a recognition that the major goal of training is a basic competency in professional and service development skills. This equips us with the conceptual and practical tools in order to learn how to learn.

Another major antecedent that may serve to impede research activity is the mental health service itself. All too often there is at best only a superficial requirement for units or services to provide data on their effectiveness. They are typically 'open-ended and non-dynamic', with no obvious relationship between the phases of input, process and output (Krapfl, 1981). It follows that objectives have been poorly delineated, making it very difficult even to begin the evaluation process.

In terms of antecedents, we need systems which signal benefits rather than punishments for engaging in evaluation. As things stand at present, practitioners engaging in research can usually anticipate considerable personal hassle as a function of their activity. As Newnes and Mercier (1986) have pointed out, research tends to extend beyond allotted time, 'affecting work, domestic arrangements, leisure time, self-esteem, frustration tolerance and capacity to devote attention to others' (p. 20). The move towards general management principles in the NHS holds the promise of a review of these conditions, with welcome suggestions, for example, for 'merit awards' and career advancement based on service evaluation and development (Milne and Aird, 1986).

13.2 CONSEQUENCES OF RESEARCH ACTIVITY

It is one thing for these so-called 'benefit signals' to be incorporated into management thinking, and quite another to consider their relationship to what actually follows most evaluation activities. The contributors to this book have generally indicated that benefits have indeed accrued to their practice. However, as the chapters by Edwards and Gambrill illustrate, there are some tensions even within mental health disciplines. Since the reaction of one's immediate colleagues would be expected to have a particularly powerful effect on one's style of work, we can see that there may need to be a considerable shift in the basic position of some disciplines in relation to evaluation. An alternative shift that might more readily occur is for local 'teams' to cohere through mutual interest. These might well cut across disciplines and settings, providing the key ingredient of service innovation, a small, mutually supportive group (Fairweather, Sanders and Tornatzky, 1974). Some of the work reported by Milne, Edwards and Grainger in this book emerged from such a group, while many other contributors have clearly been dependent upon at least the co-operation of colleagues in other disciplines. The summary provided by Fitch (1986) illustrates the work of such a group, and its contribution to research productivity under routine service conditions.

This is a more likely scenario than the one rightly mocked by

Gale (1985), in distinguishing the research dream from the reality. He caricatured the dream in these terms: 'images of beautiful scientists in white coats making brilliant discoveries. The world applauds as the King of Sweden hands over the Nobel prize to a distinguished yet shy recipient. The prize is a large cash sum' (p. 187). In keeping with our emphasis upon a research support group, Gale too asserts that 'research is a social process, set within a social context' (p. 196). For the dream to become a reality he believes that we need the co-operation of both colleagues and the system in which we work.

We will shortly be considering the kind of system that might be effective in making routine service research a reality. Before closing this section, though, it may be helpful to place this discussion in a wider social context, with the help of another societal 'dreamer', B.F. Skinner. In defining what is wrong with western society generally, Skinner (1986) picks out five cultural practices which he believes have undermined our sense of purpose. Most of these are highly relevant to the foregoing, including estranging workers from the consequences of their work; the maintenance of aversive control in work systems; and dependence on others for solutions to problems. Evaluative research seems to provide a way of reversing these practices, since the individual can 'see' the product of his/her work more completely, hence obtaining more 'natural reinforcement', and can also generate more control over the work system. Workers do not have to depend entirely on others for advice on how best to work, but can learn to generate their own solutions and consequences. This kind of shift in routine practice is funda-mental, according to Skinner, because it puts us back on our evolutionary rails. It resumes the kind of relationship between 'antecedent', 'behaviour' and 'consequence' that served to shape up our society from the beginning. It gets us interested in our work, rather than being sabotaging, stubborn or sick.

13.3 SELF-MANAGEMENT FOR THE SCIENTIST?

In this final section we will draw the preceding points into the consideration of a basic model. This model is what Skinner and other behaviourists would call 'self-management'. The term refers to the ways in which we can influence our environment so that it in turn influences us. It is rational, everyday behaviour in that it has developed to increase the likelihood of benefit and to reduce the chance of an unpleasant reaction.

In terms of the behaviour which we are interested in making an everyday occurrence — service evaluation — it means that we need to consider the kinds of antecedents and consequences mentioned earlier. However, we should consider them from the perspective of active agents, carefully manipulating how they control our research activities.

The best illustration of this 'scientist self-management' model appears to be the one described by Krapfl (1981), in which inputs, processes and outputs are related to one another in a developmental way. At the level of the individual practitioner-scientist, this model offers a framework for skilful self-management, since it requires us to see the broader consequences of our work and encourages us to monitor our progress towards certain goals. It is conceivable that adherence to the essence of this model will permit individuals to pursue service evaluation, even when the wider context is lacking in any such 'management'. From my own experience this has almost always been the position, as exemplified by Chapter 2. Indeed, from what we know of mental health service management, it must have been the case that most practitioner-scientists, including those who have contributed to this book, have survived through such self-management.

It is tempting to suggest a contrasting model, based on management as more traditionally construed. On such a basis we would be arguing for changes in the whole system as a precondition for changes in the way we work, as indeed Mechanic (1986) has done in a prospective view of service development in mental health. However, such a contrast would deny the essential continuity between individuals and their work systems. Practitioner-scientists must inevitably effect this system to greater or lesser degrees. It is therefore a case of unifying the traditional role of managers working with larger units of the system ('administrators', 'general managers', 'consultants') with those whose role spreads 'management' through more confined areas.

One way of illustrating the connection between the two overlapping forms of management comes from the work of social ecologists, since they have repeatedly shown the need to expand evaluation from a consideration of individuals (therapists and patients) to the broader assessment of social-environmental systems (e.g. Willems, 1973; Campbell, Steenberger, Smith and Stucky, 1982). Latterly there have been signs of a trend towards embedding individual-level evaluations into broader frameworks that necessarily incorporate those designated as service managers (see, for example, Finney and Moos, 1984). Christian (1984) has shown that such a framework can be put into operation successfully. He indicates that success necessarily depends upon careful attention to a systematic 'package' of interventions. In contrast, he believes that piecemeal changes are usually doomed. Consider a recent example from our local hospital for people with a mental handicap. An expensive speech synthesiser was introduced to help two clients. Such were the personal consequences of this innovation (e.g. ridicule from other clients) that the clients used the apparatus to signal that they wanted it taken away! Such resource allocation need not be totally wasteful if we can derive valuable principles about the change process. In this present example we could extend the parallel to include the likely futility of bringing in expensive people to work in systems where neither they nor their managers have ways of procuring successful change.

It is conceivable, if optimistic, that this trend towards broader evaluation will start to draw managers into rational organisational change because of the even wider political and social pressures (e.g. cost–benefit analyses; accountability). On this view the practitioner-scientist will be able to exert more self-management and will increasingly be 'locked' into a service evaluation role. Of course, this progression depends upon another rather unlikely trend, one in which important political and financial decisions are related to objective data concerning a programme's effectiveness (Stolz, 1981). We are therefore thrust back on the self-management model as the most practicable option, given present conditions.

Times inevitably change. At the moment innovations and the mental health services are rarely influenced by evaluation at all. This runs contrary to the belief that research is twice blest: it blesseth the experimenter and the experimented-upon (Rashkis, 1961). Davis and Salasin (1983) have shown how the blessing is at best only bestowed upon the researcher. They found that only 5 per cent of 600 references on evaluation pertained to utilisation, and of 1,200 references on utilisation there were only 2.5 per cent concerned with evaluation. As they point out, 'it is as difficult to see how planned change can be carried out without evaluation as it is to understand how evaluation can realise its potential without consideration of planned change' (p. 386).

Provided that the rare, self-managing practitioner-scientists continue to use the evaluation model reflexively, then they should survive. As times change they may well be provided with the kind of comprehensive, service evaluation system they require, if their style of work is to prove optimally beneficial. Better still, they will provide their managers with an acceptable and rational problem-solving model, one that becomes an integral process in the invention of better mental health services. Only then will research be truly 'twice blest'.

ACKNOWLEDGEMENTS

I am grateful to Valerie Elliott for the speech synthesiser example, and to Judy Milne for helping with the flow of the chapter.

REFERENCES

Barlow, D.H., Hayes, S.C. and Nelson, R.O. (1984) *The Scientist–Practitioner*, Pergamon Press, New York

Campbell, D.E., Steenberger, B.N., Smith, T.W. and Stucky, R.J. (1982) 'An Ecological Systems Approach to Evaluation', *Evaluation Review*, 6, pp. 625-48

Christian, W.P. (1984) 'A Case Study in the Programming and Maintenance of Institutional Change', *Journal of Organizational Behaviour Management*, 5, pp. 99-153

Davis, H.R. and Salasin, S.E. (1983) 'The Utilization of Evaluation', in: E.L. Struening and M.B. Brewer (eds), *Handbook of Evaluation Research*, Sage, London

Fairweather, G.W., Sanders, D.H. and Tornatzky, L.G. (1974) *Creating Change in Mental Health Organizations*, Pergamon Press, New York

Finney, J.W. and Moos, R.H. (1984) 'Environmental Assessment and Evaluation Research', *Evaluation and Programme Planning*, 7, pp. 151-67

Fitch, M. (1986) 'Peterborough Psychological Research Group: a 3-year Follow-up', *Clinical Psychology Forum*, 1, pp. 31-6

Gale, A. (1985) 'On Doing Research: the Dream and the Reality', *Journal of Family Therapy*, 7, pp. 187-211

Hersen, M. and Barlow, D.H. (1976) *Single Case Experimental Designs: Strategies for Studying Behavior Change*, Pergamon Press, New York

Kazdin, A.E., Kratochwill, T.R. and Vandenbos, G.R. (1986) 'Beyond Clinical Trials: Generalizing from Research to Practice', *Professional Psychology: Research and Practice, 17*, pp. 391-8

Krapfl, J. (1981) 'Behaviour Management in State Mental Health Systems', *Organizational Behaviour Management, 3*, pp. 91-105

Mechanic, D. (1986) 'The Challenge of Chronic Mental Illness', *Hospital and Community Psychiatry, 37*, pp. 891-6

Milne, D.L. and Aird, B. (1986) 'Management, Motivation and Monitoring', *Health and Social Services Journal*, 16 January, pp. 78-9

Newnes, C. and Mercier, C. (1986) 'Psychotherapy Research in the Context of a District Clinical Psychology Service', *Clinical Psychology Forum, 5*, pp. 17-20

Rashkis, H.A. (1961) 'The Research Community', *Archives of General Psychiatry, 5*, pp. 88-96

Skinner, B.F. (1986) 'What is Wrong with Daily Life in the Western World?', *American Psychologist, 41*, pp. 568-74

Stolz, S.B. (1981) 'Adoption of Innovation from Applied Behavioural Research: 'Does Anybody Care?', *Journal of Applied Behavior Analysis, 14*, pp. 491-505

Willems, E.P. (1973) 'Go Ye Into all the World and Modify Behaviour: An Ecologist's View', *Representative Research in Social Psychology, 4*, pp. 93-105

Printed and bound by CPI Group (UK) Ltd, Croydon, CR0 4YY

22/10/2024

01777615-0005

278

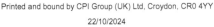

Index